Physical Wellness Unleashed

Discover the Keys to a Vibrant and Healthy Life

Wilona Floyd

The presentation of the information is without
contract or any type of guarantee assurance. The
trademarks that are used are without any consent,
and the publication of the trademark is without
permission or backing by the trademark owner. All
trademarks and brands within this book are for
clarifying purposes only and are the owned by the
owners themselves, not affiliated with this document.

Table of Contents

Chapter 1

Introduction to Physical Wellness

Understanding Physical Wellness

Physical wellness is a multifaceted concept that extends beyond the mere absence of illness. It encompasses a state of well-being where the body functions optimally, allowing individuals to engage in daily activities with vigor and vitality. At its core, physical wellness is about nurturing the body through a balanced lifestyle that includes proper nutrition, regular physical activity, adequate rest, and mental well-being. Understanding this holistic approach is crucial for anyone seeking to enhance their quality of life.

The journey to physical wellness begins with self-awareness. Recognizing the current state of one's health and identifying areas for improvement is the first step. This involves assessing dietary habits, exercise routines, sleep patterns, and stress levels. By taking stock of these elements, individuals can gain insight into how their lifestyle choices impact their overall health. This self-assessment serves as a foundation for setting realistic and achievable wellness goals.

Nutrition plays a pivotal role in physical wellness. The body requires a variety of nutrients to function effectively, and a balanced diet ensures that these needs are met. Consuming a diverse range of foods, including fruits, vegetables, whole grains, lean proteins, and healthy fats, provides the essential vitamins and minerals necessary for optimal health. It's important to understand that nutrition is not about restrictive dieting but about making informed choices that support the body's needs. By focusing on nutrient-dense foods, individuals can fuel their bodies for peak performance.

Physical activity is another cornerstone of physical wellness. Regular exercise not only strengthens the body but also enhances mental health by releasing endorphins, which are natural mood elevators. Engaging in a variety of physical activities, such as aerobic exercises, strength training, and flexibility exercises, ensures a well-rounded fitness regimen. It's essential to find activities that are enjoyable and sustainable, as consistency is key to reaping the benefits of exercise. Whether it's a brisk walk, a yoga session, or a weightlifting routine, the goal is to keep the body moving and the heart pumping.

Rest and recovery are often overlooked aspects of physical wellness. The body needs time to repair and rejuvenate, and adequate sleep is crucial for this process. Sleep deprivation can lead to a host of health issues, including weakened immunity, impaired cognitive function, and increased stress levels. Prioritizing sleep by establishing a regular sleep schedule and creating a restful environment can significantly impact overall well-being. Additionally, incorporating relaxation techniques such as meditation or deep breathing exercises can help manage stress and promote mental clarity.

The mind-body connection is an integral part of physical wellness. Mental health and physical health are deeply intertwined, and nurturing one often benefits the other. Stress, anxiety, and depression can manifest physically, leading to symptoms such as fatigue, headaches, and muscle tension. Conversely, physical ailments can affect mental health, creating a cycle that can be challenging to break. By practicing mindfulness and stress management techniques, individuals can cultivate a sense of balance and harmony between the mind and body.

Setting realistic wellness goals is essential for maintaining motivation and achieving long-term success. Goals should be specific, measurable, attainable, relevant, and time-bound (SMART). For example, instead of setting a vague goal to "get fit," one might aim to "exercise for 30 minutes, five days a week." Breaking down larger goals into smaller, manageable steps can make the process less daunting and more achievable. Celebrating small victories along the way can also boost confidence and reinforce positive behaviors.

Overcoming common barriers to physical wellness requires determination and creativity. Time constraints, lack of motivation, and limited resources are challenges that many individuals face. However, by prioritizing wellness and finding innovative solutions, these obstacles can be overcome. For instance, incorporating short bursts of activity throughout the day, preparing healthy meals in advance, and seeking support from friends or wellness communities can help maintain momentum and commitment.

Building a supportive environment is crucial for sustaining physical wellness. Surrounding oneself with positive influences, whether it's family, friends, or a community of like-minded individuals, can provide encouragement and accountability. Sharing wellness goals with others and engaging in group activities can foster a sense of camaraderie and motivation. Additionally, creating a physical space that promotes health, such as a home gym or a designated area for relaxation, can reinforce wellness habits.

Understanding physical wellness is a lifelong journey that requires continuous learning and adaptation. As individuals progress on their wellness path, they may encounter new challenges and opportunities for growth. Staying informed about the latest health research and trends can provide valuable insights and inspiration. Embracing change and being open to new experiences can lead to personal growth and a deeper understanding of what it means to be truly well.

The Importance of a Holistic Approach

Embracing a holistic approach to physical wellness is akin to weaving a tapestry where each thread contributes to the overall picture of health. This perspective acknowledges that the body, mind, and spirit are interconnected, and that true wellness arises from nurturing all aspects of oneself. By considering the whole person rather than focusing solely on physical symptoms or isolated goals, individuals can achieve a more profound and lasting sense of well-being.

The concept of holism in wellness is rooted in the understanding that every part of the body is interdependent. For instance, emotional stress can manifest physically, leading to ailments such as headaches or digestive issues. Conversely, physical discomfort can affect mental health, resulting in anxiety or depression. Recognizing these connections allows individuals to address the root causes of health issues rather than merely treating symptoms. This comprehensive approach fosters a deeper awareness of how lifestyle choices impact overall health.

One of the key elements of a holistic approach is the integration of various wellness practices that cater to different dimensions of health. Nutrition, exercise, mental health, and spiritual well-being all play vital roles in this framework. By incorporating diverse practices, individuals can create a balanced lifestyle that supports their unique needs. For example, combining a nutritious diet with regular physical activity and mindfulness exercises can enhance both physical and mental health, leading to a more harmonious existence.

Nutrition is a cornerstone of holistic wellness, as it provides the body with the essential nutrients needed for optimal function. A diet rich in whole, unprocessed foods supports not only physical health but also mental clarity and emotional stability. By focusing on nutrient-dense foods, individuals can fuel their bodies and minds, promoting energy and vitality. It's important to listen to the body's signals and adjust dietary choices accordingly, as each person's nutritional needs may vary.

Physical activity is another crucial component of a holistic approach. Regular exercise not only strengthens the body but also boosts mood and cognitive function. Engaging in a variety of activities, such as cardiovascular exercises, strength training, and flexibility workouts, ensures a well-rounded fitness regimen. The key is to find activities that are enjoyable and sustainable, as this encourages consistency and long-term commitment. Exercise can also serve as a form of meditation, allowing individuals to connect with their bodies and release stress.

Mental health is an integral part of holistic wellness, as the mind and body are inextricably linked. Practices such as mindfulness, meditation, and deep breathing can help manage stress and promote emotional balance. By cultivating a positive mindset and developing coping strategies, individuals can enhance their resilience and overall well-being. It's essential to prioritize mental health and seek support when needed, as emotional well-being is a vital component of a holistic lifestyle.

Spiritual well-being, though often overlooked, is a significant aspect of holistic wellness. This dimension involves finding meaning and purpose in life, which can be achieved through various practices such as meditation, prayer, or spending time in nature. Spirituality is a deeply personal experience, and individuals are encouraged to explore what resonates with them. By nurturing the spirit, individuals can cultivate a sense of inner peace and fulfillment, which contributes to overall wellness.

A holistic approach also emphasizes the importance of preventive care and self-awareness. By regularly monitoring one's health and making informed choices, individuals can prevent potential health issues before they arise. This proactive mindset encourages individuals to take responsibility for their well-being and make conscious decisions that support their health goals. Regular check-ups, screenings, and self-assessments are essential components of preventive care, as they provide valuable insights into one's health status.

Building a supportive environment is crucial for sustaining a holistic lifestyle. Surrounding oneself with positive influences, whether it's family, friends, or a community of like-minded individuals, can provide encouragement and accountability. Sharing wellness goals with others and engaging in group activities can foster a sense of camaraderie and motivation. Additionally, creating a physical space that promotes health, such as a home gym or a designated area for relaxation, can reinforce wellness habits.

The journey to holistic wellness is a continuous process of growth and self-discovery. As individuals progress on their wellness path, they may encounter new challenges and opportunities for learning. Staying informed about the latest health research and trends can provide valuable insights and inspiration. Embracing change and being open to new experiences can lead to personal growth and a deeper understanding of what it means to be truly well.

Setting Realistic Wellness Goals

Embarking on a wellness journey requires a clear vision and a roadmap to guide you along the way. Setting realistic wellness goals is an essential step in this process, as it provides direction and motivation while ensuring that your aspirations are achievable and sustainable. By establishing well-defined objectives, you can create a structured plan that aligns with your unique needs and lifestyle, ultimately leading to lasting improvements in your overall well-being.

The first step in setting realistic wellness goals is to conduct a thorough self-assessment. This involves evaluating your current health status, identifying areas for improvement, and considering any limitations or constraints you may face. Reflect on your dietary habits, exercise routines, sleep patterns, and stress levels, as these factors play a significant role in your overall wellness. By gaining a comprehensive understanding of your starting point, you can set goals that are both challenging and attainable.

Once you have a clear picture of your current state, it's time to define your wellness goals. These objectives should be specific, measurable, attainable, relevant, and time-bound (SMART). Specific goals provide clarity and focus, while measurable goals allow you to track your progress and celebrate achievements. Attainable goals ensure that your aspirations are realistic and within reach, while relevant goals align with your values and priorities. Finally, time-bound goals create a sense of urgency and help you stay on track.

For example, instead of setting a vague goal to "eat healthier," you might aim to "incorporate at least five servings of fruits and vegetables into your daily diet." This goal is specific, measurable, and relevant to your overall wellness. By breaking down larger goals into smaller, manageable steps, you can make the process less daunting and more achievable. This approach also allows you to build momentum and confidence as you progress on your wellness journey.

It's important to recognize that wellness goals are not one-size-fits-all. Each individual's needs and circumstances are unique, and your goals should reflect your personal preferences and lifestyle. Consider factors such as your work schedule, family commitments, and social obligations when setting your objectives. By tailoring your goals to fit your life, you can create a plan that is both practical and sustainable.

Flexibility is another crucial aspect of setting realistic wellness goals. Life is unpredictable, and circumstances may change over time. It's essential to remain adaptable and open to adjusting your goals as needed. If you encounter obstacles or setbacks, don't be discouraged. Instead, view these challenges as opportunities for growth and learning. By maintaining a flexible mindset, you can navigate the ups and downs of your wellness journey with resilience and determination.

Accountability is a powerful tool for achieving wellness goals. Sharing your objectives with a trusted friend, family member, or wellness coach can provide support and encouragement. Having someone to hold you accountable can help you stay committed and motivated, especially during challenging times. Additionally, tracking your progress through journals, apps, or other tools can provide valuable insights and reinforce positive behaviors.

Celebrating milestones and achievements is an essential part of the goal-setting process. Recognizing your accomplishments, no matter how small, can boost your confidence and motivation. Take the time to acknowledge your progress and reward yourself for your hard work and dedication. This positive reinforcement can help you stay focused and committed to your long-term wellness goals.

As you work towards your objectives, it's important to maintain a balanced perspective. Wellness is a lifelong journey, and progress may not always be linear. There may be times when you experience setbacks or plateaus, but these moments are a natural part of the process. By focusing on the bigger picture and maintaining a positive attitude, you can overcome challenges and continue moving forward.

Incorporating mindfulness and self-reflection into your goal-setting process can enhance your overall experience. Take the time to regularly assess your progress and evaluate whether your goals still align with your values and priorities. This practice can help you stay connected to your intentions and ensure that your wellness journey remains meaningful and fulfilling.

Overcoming Common Barriers

Embarking on a journey towards physical wellness is a commendable endeavor, yet it often comes with its fair share of obstacles. These barriers can manifest in various forms, from time constraints and lack of motivation to financial limitations and environmental factors. Understanding and overcoming these common challenges is crucial for maintaining momentum and achieving long-term success in your wellness journey.

One of the most prevalent barriers to physical wellness is time. In today's fast-paced world, many individuals struggle to find the time to prioritize their health amidst work, family, and social commitments. However, it's important to recognize that wellness is an investment in oneself, and making time for it is essential. To overcome this barrier, consider integrating wellness activities into your daily routine. For instance, you might incorporate short bursts of physical activity throughout the day, such as taking the stairs instead of the elevator or going for a brisk walk during lunch breaks. Additionally, meal prepping on weekends can save time during the week and ensure that you have healthy options readily available.

Lack of motivation is another common hurdle that many individuals face. It's natural for motivation to ebb and flow, but finding ways to stay inspired is key to maintaining consistency. Setting clear, achievable goals and tracking your progress can provide a sense of purpose and direction. Visualizing the benefits of your efforts, such as improved energy levels or enhanced mood, can also serve as a powerful motivator. Surrounding yourself with supportive individuals, whether it's friends, family, or a wellness community, can provide encouragement and accountability. Sharing your goals with others and celebrating milestones together can foster a sense of camaraderie and motivation.

Financial constraints can also pose a challenge to achieving physical wellness. Gym memberships, organic foods, and wellness programs can be costly, but there are plenty of budget-friendly alternatives. Exploring free or low-cost resources, such as online workout videos, community fitness classes, or local parks, can provide opportunities for physical activity without breaking the bank. When it comes to nutrition, focusing on whole, unprocessed foods and buying in bulk can help stretch your budget. Planning meals around seasonal produce and taking advantage of sales can also make healthy eating more affordable.

Environmental factors, such as living in an area with limited access to recreational facilities or healthy food options, can also impact one's ability to pursue wellness goals. In such cases, creativity and resourcefulness are essential. If outdoor spaces are limited, consider creating a home workout space with minimal equipment, such as resistance bands or bodyweight exercises. For those with limited access to fresh produce, exploring community gardens or farmers' markets can provide alternative sources of nutritious foods. Additionally, advocating for improved wellness resources in your community can lead to positive changes and increased access for all.

Stress and mental health challenges can also act as barriers to physical wellness. High stress levels can lead to emotional eating, lack of motivation, and disrupted sleep patterns, all of which can hinder progress. Incorporating stress management techniques, such as mindfulness, meditation, or deep breathing exercises, can help alleviate stress and promote mental clarity. Prioritizing self-care and seeking support from mental health professionals when needed can also enhance emotional well-being and support your wellness journey.

Another common barrier is the fear of failure or perfectionism. Many individuals set unrealistic expectations for themselves, leading to feelings of frustration and disappointment when they fall short. It's important to remember that wellness is a lifelong journey, and progress may not always be linear. Embracing a growth mindset and viewing setbacks as opportunities for learning and growth can help build resilience and perseverance. Celebrating small victories and acknowledging your efforts, regardless of the outcome, can boost confidence and motivation.

Social and cultural influences can also impact one's ability to pursue wellness goals. Peer pressure, cultural norms, and societal expectations can create obstacles to making healthy choices. Navigating these influences requires self-awareness and assertiveness. Setting boundaries and communicating your wellness goals to others can help create a supportive environment. Seeking out like-minded individuals or communities that share your values can also provide a sense of belonging and encouragement.

Finally, it's important to recognize that overcoming barriers to physical wellness is a dynamic and ongoing process. As life circumstances change, new challenges may arise, requiring adaptability and flexibility. Staying informed about the latest wellness trends and research can provide valuable insights and inspiration. Embracing change and being open to new experiences can lead to personal growth and a deeper understanding of what it means to be truly well.

Building a Supportive Environment

Creating a supportive environment is a crucial element in the pursuit of physical wellness. It acts as the foundation upon which healthy habits are built and sustained. A nurturing environment not only provides the necessary resources and encouragement but also fosters a sense of belonging and motivation. By surrounding yourself with positive influences and making strategic adjustments to your surroundings, you can significantly enhance your ability to achieve and maintain your wellness goals.

The first step in building a supportive environment is to assess your current surroundings and identify areas that may need improvement. Consider the physical spaces where you spend most of your time, such as your home, workplace, and community. Evaluate whether these environments promote or hinder your wellness efforts. For instance, a cluttered and disorganized home may contribute to stress and make it difficult to focus on healthy habits. Similarly, a workplace that lacks access to nutritious food options or opportunities for physical activity may pose challenges to maintaining a balanced lifestyle.

Once you have identified potential barriers, take proactive steps to create a more conducive environment for wellness. In your home, consider designating specific areas for activities that support your health goals. For example, create a dedicated space for exercise, meditation, or meal preparation. This can help establish a routine and make it easier to incorporate wellness practices into your daily life. Additionally, organizing your living space and reducing clutter can promote a sense of calm and focus, allowing you to concentrate on your wellness journey.

In the workplace, advocate for changes that support a healthier lifestyle. This might include requesting access to healthier food options in the cafeteria, organizing group fitness activities, or encouraging walking meetings. If possible, personalize your workspace to include elements that promote well-being, such as ergonomic furniture, plants, or motivational quotes. By taking initiative and collaborating with colleagues, you can create a more supportive work environment that aligns with your wellness goals.

Community plays a significant role in building a supportive environment. Engaging with like-minded individuals who share your wellness aspirations can provide encouragement, accountability, and inspiration. Seek out local wellness groups, fitness classes, or online communities where you can connect with others who are on a similar journey. Participating in group activities or challenges can foster a sense of camaraderie and motivation, making it easier to stay committed to your goals.

Social support is another critical component of a supportive environment. Surround yourself with friends and family members who encourage and support your wellness efforts. Share your goals with them and communicate how they can help you stay on track. Whether it's joining you for a workout, preparing healthy meals together, or simply offering words of encouragement, having a strong support network can make a significant difference in your ability to achieve and maintain your wellness objectives.

In addition to social support, consider seeking guidance from wellness professionals, such as nutritionists, personal trainers, or mental health counselors. These experts can provide valuable insights, personalized advice, and accountability, helping you navigate challenges and make informed decisions. By building a team of professionals who understand your goals and needs, you can enhance your ability to achieve lasting success.

Creating a supportive environment also involves setting boundaries and managing external influences that may hinder your progress. This might include limiting exposure to negative influences, such as social media or individuals who discourage your wellness efforts. Establishing clear boundaries and prioritizing your well-being can help you stay focused and committed to your goals.

It's important to recognize that building a supportive environment is an ongoing process that requires continuous evaluation and adaptation. As your wellness journey evolves, your needs and circumstances may change, necessitating adjustments to your environment. Regularly assess your surroundings and make necessary changes to ensure that they continue to support your goals.

Incorporating mindfulness and self-reflection into your routine can enhance your ability to create and maintain a supportive environment. Take the time to regularly evaluate your progress and consider how your environment impacts your wellness journey. This practice can help you stay connected to your intentions and ensure that your surroundings align with your values and priorities.

Chapter 2

Nourishing Your Body

The Fundamentals of Nutrition

Nutrition is the cornerstone of physical wellness, serving as the fuel that powers our bodies and minds. Understanding the fundamentals of nutrition is essential for making informed choices that support overall health and vitality. By grasping the basic principles of nutrition, individuals can create balanced diets that meet their unique needs and promote long-term well-being.

At the heart of nutrition are macronutrients: carbohydrates, proteins, and fats. These nutrients provide the energy and building blocks necessary for bodily functions. Carbohydrates are the body's primary energy source, found in foods like grains, fruits, and vegetables. They are broken down into glucose, which fuels our cells and supports brain function. It's important to choose complex carbohydrates, such as whole grains and legumes, which provide sustained energy and are rich in fiber, aiding digestion and promoting satiety.

Proteins are vital for growth, repair, and maintenance of tissues. They are composed of amino acids, some of which are essential and must be obtained through diet. Sources of protein include meat, fish, dairy, legumes, and nuts. Incorporating a variety of protein sources ensures a complete amino acid profile, supporting muscle health and immune function. For those following plant-based diets, combining different plant proteins, such as beans and rice, can provide all essential amino acids.

Fats, often misunderstood, are crucial for overall health. They serve as a concentrated energy source, support cell structure, and aid in the absorption of fat-soluble vitamins. Healthy fats, such as those found in avocados, nuts, seeds, and olive oil, should be prioritized. These unsaturated fats can improve heart health and reduce inflammation. Conversely, trans fats and excessive saturated fats, commonly found in processed foods, should be limited due to their association with heart disease.

Micronutrients, including vitamins and minerals, are equally important, though required in smaller amounts. They play critical roles in various bodily processes, from bone health to immune function. A diverse diet rich in fruits, vegetables, whole grains, and lean proteins typically provides the necessary micronutrients. However, certain populations, such as pregnant women or the elderly, may require supplements to meet their specific needs. Consulting with a healthcare professional can help determine if supplementation is necessary.

Hydration is another fundamental aspect of nutrition. Water is essential for maintaining bodily functions, regulating temperature, and transporting nutrients. Dehydration can lead to fatigue, impaired cognitive function, and other health issues. It's important to consume adequate fluids throughout the day, with water being the preferred choice. While individual hydration needs vary, a general guideline is to drink at least eight 8-ounce glasses of water daily, adjusting for factors such as activity level and climate.

Understanding portion sizes and practicing mindful eating can further enhance nutritional habits. In today's fast-paced world, it's easy to overlook portion control, leading to overconsumption and weight gain. Being mindful of portion sizes and listening to hunger cues can help maintain a healthy weight and prevent overeating. Mindful eating involves savoring each bite, paying attention to flavors and textures, and recognizing when you're satisfied, rather than eating until you're full.

Meal planning and preparation are practical strategies for maintaining a balanced diet. By planning meals in advance, individuals can ensure they have nutritious options readily available, reducing the temptation to opt for convenience foods. Preparing meals at home allows for greater control over ingredients and portion sizes, promoting healthier eating habits. Batch cooking and using leftovers creatively can save time and effort, making it easier to stick to a nutritious diet.

Navigating food labels is an essential skill for making informed dietary choices. Food labels provide valuable information about the nutritional content of packaged foods, including serving size, calorie count, and nutrient breakdown. Understanding how to read and interpret these labels can help individuals make healthier choices and avoid foods high in added sugars, sodium, and unhealthy fats. Paying attention to ingredient lists can also reveal the presence of additives or allergens.

Cultural and personal preferences play a significant role in shaping dietary habits. Embracing cultural diversity in food choices can enhance the enjoyment of meals and provide a wide range of nutrients. Exploring different cuisines and incorporating a variety of flavors and ingredients can make healthy eating more exciting and sustainable. It's important to find a balance between honoring cultural traditions and making choices that support overall health.

The fundamentals of nutrition also involve recognizing the impact of dietary patterns on long-term health. Diets rich in whole, unprocessed foods are associated with a reduced risk of chronic diseases, such as heart disease, diabetes, and certain cancers. Conversely, diets high in processed foods, added sugars, and unhealthy fats can contribute to the development of these conditions. By prioritizing whole foods and minimizing processed options, individuals can support their long-term health and well-being.

Incorporating these nutritional principles into daily life requires commitment and adaptability. As individuals progress on their wellness journey, they may encounter challenges and opportunities for growth. Staying informed about the latest nutrition research and trends can provide valuable insights and inspiration. Embracing change and being open to new experiences can lead to personal growth and a deeper understanding of what it means to be truly well.

Superfoods for Optimal Health

Superfoods have captured the imagination of health enthusiasts around the globe, promising a bounty of nutrients packed into every bite. These nutrient-dense foods are celebrated for their potential to enhance health and vitality, offering a natural way to boost the body's defenses and support overall well-being. While the term "superfood" is not a scientific classification, it serves as a convenient label for foods that are exceptionally rich in vitamins, minerals, antioxidants, and other beneficial compounds.

One of the most renowned superfoods is the humble blueberry. These small, vibrant berries are bursting with antioxidants, particularly anthocyanins, which give them their deep blue hue. Antioxidants play a crucial role in neutralizing free radicals, unstable molecules that can cause cellular damage and contribute to aging and disease. Regular consumption of blueberries has been linked to improved brain health, reduced inflammation, and a lower risk of heart disease. Their sweet, tangy flavor makes them a versatile addition to smoothies, yogurt, or salads.

Kale, often hailed as a nutritional powerhouse, is another superfood that has gained popularity in recent years. This leafy green is packed with vitamins A, C, and K, as well as calcium, iron, and fiber. Its high nutrient content supports bone health, boosts the immune system, and aids in digestion. Kale's versatility allows it to be enjoyed in a variety of dishes, from salads and soups to smoothies and stir-fries. For those who find its flavor too robust, massaging the leaves with a bit of olive oil and lemon juice can soften its texture and mellow its taste.

Quinoa, a staple in many plant-based diets, is a complete protein, meaning it contains all nine essential amino acids. This ancient grain is also rich in fiber, magnesium, and manganese, making it an excellent choice for supporting muscle function, digestion, and bone health. Quinoa's mild, nutty flavor and fluffy texture make it a versatile base for salads, bowls, and side dishes. Its quick cooking time and adaptability to various cuisines have contributed to its widespread appeal.

Chia seeds, though tiny, pack a powerful nutritional punch. These seeds are an excellent source of omega-3 fatty acids, fiber, and protein. Omega-3s are essential fats that support heart health, reduce inflammation, and promote brain function. Chia seeds' unique ability to absorb liquid and form a gel-like consistency makes them a popular ingredient in puddings, smoothies, and baked goods. Their neutral flavor allows them to be easily incorporated into a variety of recipes without altering the taste.

Avocados, with their creamy texture and rich flavor, are a beloved superfood known for their heart-healthy monounsaturated fats. These fats help lower bad cholesterol levels and reduce the risk of heart disease. Avocados are also a good source of potassium, which supports healthy blood pressure levels. Their versatility extends beyond guacamole; they can be sliced onto toast, blended into smoothies, or used as a substitute for butter in baking.

Turmeric, a vibrant yellow spice commonly used in Indian cuisine, has gained recognition for its anti-inflammatory properties. Curcumin, the active compound in turmeric, has been studied for its potential to reduce inflammation and support joint health. Incorporating turmeric into the diet can be as simple as adding it to soups, stews, or rice dishes. For enhanced absorption, it's often paired with black pepper, which contains piperine, a compound that increases curcumin's bioavailability.

Salmon, a fatty fish rich in omega-3 fatty acids, is another superfood that supports heart and brain health. These essential fats have been shown to reduce the risk of heart disease, improve cognitive function, and support mental health. Salmon is also an excellent source of high-quality protein and vitamin D, which are important for muscle maintenance and bone health. Grilled, baked, or poached, salmon can be enjoyed in a variety of dishes, from salads to pasta.

Sweet potatoes, with their vibrant orange flesh, are a nutrient-dense root vegetable rich in beta-carotene, a precursor to vitamin A. This vitamin is essential for maintaining healthy vision, skin, and immune function. Sweet potatoes are also a good source of fiber, which supports digestive health and helps regulate blood sugar levels. Their natural sweetness makes them a versatile ingredient in both savory and sweet dishes, from roasted sides to pies and casseroles.

Incorporating superfoods into your diet doesn't require a complete overhaul of your eating habits. Instead, consider adding these nutrient-rich foods to your existing meals and snacks. For example, sprinkle chia seeds on your morning cereal, toss a handful of blueberries into your yogurt, or add a few slices of avocado to your sandwich. By gradually introducing superfoods into your diet, you can enjoy their health benefits without feeling overwhelmed.

It's important to remember that no single food can provide all the nutrients your body needs. A balanced diet that includes a variety of foods is essential for optimal health. While superfoods can enhance your nutritional intake, they should be part of a diverse and well-rounded diet. Additionally, focusing on whole, minimally processed foods and practicing mindful eating can further support your wellness journey.

As you explore the world of superfoods, be open to trying new flavors and ingredients. Experimenting with different recipes and cooking methods can make healthy eating an enjoyable and rewarding experience. By embracing the abundance of nutrient-dense foods available, you can nourish your body and support your overall well-being.

Meal Planning and Preparation

Meal planning and preparation are essential skills for anyone seeking to maintain a balanced and nutritious diet. These practices not only save time and reduce stress but also ensure that healthy meals are readily available, making it easier to adhere to dietary goals. By taking a proactive approach to meal planning and preparation, individuals can enjoy a variety of delicious and nourishing meals while minimizing food waste and maximizing efficiency.

The first step in effective meal planning is to assess your dietary needs and preferences. Consider any specific nutritional goals you may have, such as increasing protein intake, reducing sugar consumption, or incorporating more plant-based meals. Understanding your unique needs will guide your meal planning process and help you create a balanced and satisfying menu. Additionally, take into account any dietary restrictions or allergies, as well as the preferences of other household members, to ensure that everyone can enjoy the meals you prepare.

Once you have a clear understanding of your dietary needs, it's time to create a meal plan. Start by selecting a variety of recipes that align with your goals and preferences. Aim for a diverse menu that includes a range of flavors, textures, and nutrients. This not only keeps meals interesting but also ensures that you're getting a wide array of essential vitamins and minerals. Consider incorporating seasonal produce, as it tends to be fresher, more flavorful, and often more affordable.

When planning your meals, think about how you can repurpose ingredients across multiple dishes. For example, if you're making a roasted chicken for dinner, consider using the leftovers in a salad or sandwich the next day. This approach not only saves time and effort but also reduces food waste. Additionally, plan for meals that can be easily scaled up or down, allowing you to adjust portion sizes based on the number of people you're serving.

With your meal plan in place, the next step is to create a detailed shopping list. A well-organized list helps streamline your grocery shopping experience and ensures that you have all the necessary ingredients on hand. Group items by category, such as produce, dairy, and pantry staples, to make your shopping trip more efficient. As you shop, be mindful of portion sizes and expiration dates to avoid over-purchasing and minimize waste.

Meal preparation, or "meal prep," involves preparing ingredients or entire meals in advance, making it easier to enjoy healthy, home-cooked meals throughout the week. Set aside a specific day or time each week for meal prep, and consider it an investment in your health and well-being. Begin by washing, chopping, and portioning ingredients, such as vegetables, proteins, and grains. Store these prepped ingredients in airtight containers in the refrigerator or freezer, making them easily accessible when it's time to cook.

Batch cooking is another effective meal prep strategy. By preparing large quantities of certain dishes, you can enjoy them throughout the week or freeze portions for later use. Soups, stews, casseroles, and grain-based dishes like quinoa or rice are ideal candidates for batch cooking. Not only does this save time, but it also ensures that you always have a nutritious meal option available, even on the busiest days.

Incorporating variety into your meal prep routine can prevent monotony and keep meals exciting. Experiment with different cuisines, spices, and cooking techniques to discover new flavors and textures. For instance, try roasting vegetables with different herbs and spices, or explore international dishes that introduce new ingredients and culinary traditions. This approach not only enhances your culinary skills but also broadens your palate and appreciation for diverse foods.

To further streamline meal preparation, consider investing in kitchen tools and appliances that can save time and effort. A slow cooker or pressure cooker can simplify the cooking process, allowing you to prepare meals with minimal hands-on time. A food processor can quickly chop, slice, or puree ingredients, while a high-quality set of knives can make prep work more efficient and enjoyable. These tools can be valuable allies in your meal prep journey, helping you create delicious and nutritious meals with ease.

Mindful eating is an important aspect of meal planning and preparation. By taking the time to savor each bite and appreciate the flavors and textures of your meals, you can enhance your dining experience and foster a deeper connection to the food you eat. Mindful eating also encourages you to listen to your body's hunger and fullness cues, promoting a healthy relationship with food and preventing overeating.

As you become more comfortable with meal planning and preparation, consider involving family members or friends in the process. Cooking together can be a fun and rewarding experience, fostering a sense of community and shared responsibility. It also provides an opportunity to teach children valuable cooking skills and instill healthy eating habits from a young age.

Finally, remember that flexibility is key to successful meal planning and preparation. Life is unpredictable, and there may be times when your plans need to be adjusted. Embrace these moments as opportunities to be creative and resourceful, whether it's improvising with ingredients you have on hand or trying a new recipe. By maintaining a flexible mindset, you can

navigate the challenges of meal planning with
confidence and ease.

Hydration The Essential Element

Water, the elixir of life, is an essential element that
sustains every cell, tissue, and organ in our bodies.
Hydration plays a pivotal role in maintaining overall
health and well-being, yet it is often overlooked in the
hustle and bustle of daily life. Understanding the
importance of hydration and incorporating it into
your wellness routine can have profound effects on
your physical and mental health.

The human body is composed of approximately 60%
water, highlighting its significance in our
physiological processes. Water acts as a medium for
chemical reactions, aids in digestion, regulates body
temperature, and facilitates the transport of nutrients
and oxygen to cells. It also plays a crucial role in
removing waste products through urine and sweat.
Without adequate hydration, these vital functions can
be compromised, leading to a range of health issues.

One of the most immediate effects of dehydration is
fatigue. Even mild dehydration can lead to feelings of
tiredness and lethargy, impacting productivity and
cognitive function. This is because water is essential
for maintaining blood volume and circulation,
ensuring that oxygen and nutrients reach the brain
and muscles. When hydration levels drop, the body
must work harder to perform these tasks, resulting in
decreased energy levels.

Cognitive performance is also closely linked to hydration status. Studies have shown that dehydration can impair concentration, memory, and mood. This is particularly concerning for individuals who require mental acuity for work or study. By maintaining optimal hydration, you can support brain function and enhance your ability to focus and process information.

Physical performance is another area where hydration plays a critical role. During exercise, the body loses water through sweat, which can lead to dehydration if not replenished. This can result in decreased endurance, increased perceived effort, and a higher risk of heat-related illnesses. Athletes and active individuals should prioritize hydration before, during, and after exercise to maintain performance and prevent dehydration-related complications.

Hydration is also essential for maintaining healthy skin. Water helps to keep the skin hydrated and supple, reducing the appearance of fine lines and wrinkles. It also supports the skin's barrier function, protecting against environmental damage and preventing moisture loss. While topical skincare products can help, adequate hydration from within is key to achieving a radiant complexion.

The digestive system relies on water to function effectively. It aids in the breakdown and absorption of nutrients, as well as the elimination of waste products. Insufficient hydration can lead to digestive issues such as constipation, as the body draws water from the colon to maintain hydration levels. Drinking enough water can help prevent these issues and support a healthy digestive tract.

Hydration needs can vary based on factors such as age, activity level, climate, and overall health. While the commonly cited guideline is to drink eight 8-ounce glasses of water per day, individual requirements may differ. A more personalized approach is to listen to your body's thirst signals and adjust your fluid intake accordingly. Additionally, monitoring the color of your urine can provide insight into your hydration status; pale yellow urine typically indicates adequate hydration.

Incorporating a variety of fluids into your diet can help meet your hydration needs. While water is the best choice, other beverages such as herbal teas, milk, and natural fruit juices can also contribute to your daily fluid intake. Be mindful of caffeinated and sugary drinks, as they can have diuretic effects and may not provide the same hydrating benefits as water.

Foods with high water content can also support hydration. Fruits and vegetables such as watermelon, cucumber, and oranges are excellent choices, as they provide both hydration and essential nutrients. Including these foods in your meals and snacks can help you stay hydrated while enjoying a diverse and balanced diet.

For those who struggle to drink enough water, there are several strategies to make hydration more appealing. Infusing water with fresh fruits, herbs, or a splash of citrus can add flavor and make it more enjoyable to drink. Carrying a reusable water bottle throughout the day serves as a visual reminder to hydrate and makes it convenient to sip water on the go. Setting hydration goals and tracking your intake can also help establish a consistent routine.

It's important to recognize the signs of dehydration and take action to address them promptly. Symptoms such as dry mouth, headache, dizziness, and dark urine can indicate that your body needs more fluids. In severe cases, dehydration can lead to more serious complications, requiring medical attention. By staying attuned to your body's signals and prioritizing hydration, you can prevent these issues and support your overall health.

Hydration is a simple yet powerful tool for enhancing well-being. By making it a priority in your daily routine, you can experience increased energy, improved cognitive function, and better physical performance. Embracing the habit of regular hydration can lead to lasting benefits, contributing to a healthier and more vibrant life.

Supplements Do You Need Them

Navigating the world of dietary supplements can be a daunting task, with countless products promising to enhance health, boost energy, and fill nutritional gaps. The question of whether supplements are necessary is one that many individuals grapple with, especially in the context of maintaining a balanced diet and healthy lifestyle. Understanding the role of supplements and determining if they are needed requires a careful examination of individual dietary habits, health goals, and specific nutritional needs.

Supplements are designed to provide nutrients that may not be consumed in sufficient quantities through diet alone. They come in various forms, including vitamins, minerals, amino acids, and herbal extracts.

While they can be beneficial in certain situations, they are not a substitute for a well-rounded diet rich in whole foods. The foundation of good nutrition lies in consuming a diverse array of fruits, vegetables, whole grains, lean proteins, and healthy fats, which provide a wide range of essential nutrients and bioactive compounds.

For some individuals, supplements may be necessary to address specific deficiencies or health conditions. For example, vitamin D is a nutrient that many people struggle to obtain in adequate amounts, particularly those living in regions with limited sunlight exposure. Vitamin D plays a crucial role in bone health, immune function, and mood regulation. In such cases, a supplement can help ensure sufficient intake and support overall health.

Similarly, individuals following a vegan or vegetarian diet may require vitamin B12 supplementation, as this vitamin is primarily found in animal products. Vitamin B12 is essential for nerve function and the production of red blood cells. Without adequate intake, individuals may experience fatigue, neurological issues, and anemia. A B12 supplement can help prevent these deficiencies and support a plant-based lifestyle.

Iron is another nutrient that may require supplementation, particularly for women of childbearing age, pregnant individuals, and those with certain medical conditions. Iron is vital for the production of hemoglobin, which carries oxygen in the blood. Iron deficiency can lead to anemia, characterized by fatigue, weakness, and impaired cognitive function. In such cases, an iron supplement can help restore optimal levels and improve overall well-being.

Calcium and magnesium are minerals that play important roles in bone health, muscle function, and nerve transmission. While they can be obtained through dietary sources such as dairy products, leafy greens, and nuts, some individuals may struggle to meet their needs through diet alone. This is particularly true for those with lactose intolerance or dietary restrictions. In these instances, a supplement can help bridge the gap and support bone and muscle health.

Omega-3 fatty acids, found in fatty fish like salmon and mackerel, are known for their anti-inflammatory properties and benefits for heart and brain health. For individuals who do not consume fish regularly, an omega-3 supplement derived from fish oil or algae can provide these essential fats and support cardiovascular and cognitive function.

While supplements can be beneficial in certain situations, it's important to approach them with caution. Not all supplements are created equal, and the quality, potency, and safety of products can vary widely. It's essential to choose reputable brands that adhere to good manufacturing practices and provide third-party testing to ensure purity and potency. Consulting with a healthcare professional or registered dietitian can help determine the appropriate dosage and ensure that supplements are used safely and effectively.

It's also important to be aware of potential interactions between supplements and medications.

Some supplements can interfere with the absorption or effectiveness of prescription drugs, leading to adverse effects. For example, high doses of vitamin K can interfere with blood-thinning medications, while certain herbal supplements may affect liver enzymes and alter drug metabolism. Always inform your healthcare provider of any supplements you are taking to avoid potential interactions and ensure safe use.

In addition to considering individual needs and potential interactions, it's crucial to evaluate the evidence supporting the use of specific supplements. While some supplements have been extensively studied and proven effective, others may lack robust scientific evidence. Be wary of products that make exaggerated claims or promise quick fixes, as these are often not supported by credible research.

Ultimately, the decision to use supplements should be based on a comprehensive assessment of dietary habits, health goals, and individual needs. For many people, a balanced diet rich in whole foods can provide the necessary nutrients without the need for supplementation. However, in certain cases, supplements can play a valuable role in supporting health and well-being.

To make informed decisions about supplements, consider the following steps: assess your dietary intake and identify any potential nutrient gaps, consult with a healthcare professional to determine if supplements are necessary, choose high-quality products from reputable brands, and monitor your response to supplementation, adjusting as needed.

Chapter 3

The Power of Movement

Types of Physical Activity

Physical activity is a cornerstone of a healthy lifestyle, offering a multitude of benefits that extend beyond physical health to encompass mental and emotional well-being. Understanding the various types of physical activity and their unique advantages can empower individuals to create a balanced and enjoyable fitness routine tailored to their needs and preferences. From aerobic exercises to strength training, flexibility work, and balance exercises, each type of activity plays a distinct role in promoting overall health.

Aerobic exercises, often referred to as cardiovascular or endurance activities, are designed to increase heart rate and improve the efficiency of the cardiovascular system. These activities include walking, running, cycling, swimming, and dancing, among others. Aerobic exercises are particularly effective for enhancing cardiovascular health, boosting lung capacity, and increasing stamina. They also play a significant role in weight management, as they burn calories and help maintain a healthy metabolism. Engaging in regular aerobic exercise can reduce the risk of chronic diseases such as heart disease, stroke, and type 2 diabetes.

For those new to aerobic exercise, starting with low-impact activities like walking or swimming can be a gentle introduction. These activities are easy on the joints and can be gradually intensified as fitness levels improve. Incorporating variety into aerobic workouts can prevent boredom and keep motivation high. For instance, alternating between cycling and dancing or exploring different walking routes can make the experience more enjoyable and sustainable.

Strength training, also known as resistance or weight training, focuses on building and maintaining muscle mass and strength. This type of exercise involves the use of weights, resistance bands, or body weight to create resistance against muscle contractions. Strength training is essential for maintaining bone density, improving joint function, and enhancing overall physical performance. It also plays a crucial role in metabolic health, as increased muscle mass can boost resting metabolic rate and aid in weight management.

Beginners can start with bodyweight exercises such as push-ups, squats, and lunges, gradually incorporating weights or resistance bands as they become more comfortable. It's important to focus on proper form and technique to prevent injury and maximize the benefits of each exercise. Working with a certified trainer or following a structured program can provide guidance and support, ensuring that strength training is both effective and safe.

Flexibility exercises are designed to improve the range of motion in the joints and lengthen muscles. Activities such as yoga, Pilates, and stretching routines fall into this category. Flexibility work is essential for maintaining mobility, preventing injury, and reducing muscle tension. It also promotes relaxation and stress relief, contributing to overall mental well-being. Regular flexibility exercises can enhance posture, balance, and coordination, making daily activities easier and more comfortable.

Incorporating flexibility exercises into a fitness routine can be as simple as dedicating a few minutes to stretching after each workout. Yoga and Pilates classes offer structured opportunities to improve flexibility while also building strength and mindfulness. These practices encourage a holistic approach to fitness, integrating physical, mental, and emotional elements.

Balance exercises are often overlooked but are crucial for maintaining stability and preventing falls, especially as we age. Activities that challenge balance include tai chi, standing on one leg, and using balance boards or stability balls. Balance exercises strengthen the core and lower body muscles, enhancing coordination and proprioception. They are particularly beneficial for older adults, athletes, and individuals recovering from injury.

Incorporating balance exercises into a fitness routine can be simple and effective. Practicing standing on one leg while brushing teeth or incorporating tai chi movements into a warm-up routine can improve balance over time. These exercises can be adapted to suit different fitness levels and can be performed almost anywhere, making them a convenient addition to any workout regimen.

In addition to these primary types of physical activity, there are numerous other forms of exercise that offer unique benefits and can be tailored to individual preferences. High-intensity interval training (HIIT) combines short bursts of intense activity with periods of rest or low-intensity exercise, providing an efficient and effective workout. HIIT is known for its ability to improve cardiovascular fitness, increase calorie burn, and enhance metabolic health in a short amount of time.

Mind-body exercises, such as tai chi and qigong, emphasize the connection between physical movement and mental focus. These practices promote relaxation, stress reduction, and mindfulness, contributing to overall well-being. They are particularly beneficial for individuals seeking a low-impact, meditative approach to fitness.

Recreational activities, such as hiking, kayaking, or playing sports, offer opportunities for physical activity in a fun and social setting. These activities provide a break from structured workouts and allow individuals to enjoy the outdoors, connect with others, and explore new environments. Engaging in recreational activities can enhance motivation and adherence to a fitness routine, as they offer variety and enjoyment.

When designing a fitness routine, it's important to consider individual goals, preferences, and lifestyle factors. A balanced approach that incorporates a mix of aerobic, strength, flexibility, and balance exercises can provide comprehensive health benefits and prevent burnout. Listening to the body and allowing for rest and recovery is also essential, as it ensures that the body can adapt and grow stronger over time.

Designing a Personalized Exercise Routine

Crafting a personalized exercise routine is akin to designing a bespoke suit; it must fit the individual perfectly, taking into account their unique goals, preferences, and lifestyle. The journey to creating an effective and enjoyable fitness plan begins with self-assessment, where one evaluates their current fitness level, health status, and personal objectives. This introspection lays the foundation for a routine that not only aligns with one's aspirations but also adapts to their daily life.

Understanding your fitness goals is the first step in this process. Are you aiming to lose weight, build muscle, increase endurance, or simply maintain overall health? Each goal requires a different approach, and recognizing what you want to achieve will guide the selection of exercises and the structure of your routine. For instance, someone focused on weight loss might prioritize cardiovascular activities, while another aiming to build muscle would incorporate more strength training.

Once goals are established, it's essential to consider personal preferences and interests. Exercise should be enjoyable, not a chore. Reflect on activities that bring joy and excitement, whether it's dancing, swimming, hiking, or playing a sport. Incorporating these into your routine increases the likelihood of adherence and long-term success. Variety is also key; mixing different types of exercises can prevent boredom and keep motivation high.

Time is a crucial factor in designing a personalized exercise routine. Assess your schedule and determine how much time you can realistically dedicate to exercise each week. Consistency is more important than duration, so even short, regular workouts can be effective. Consider breaking sessions into manageable chunks, such as 20-30 minutes, to fit seamlessly into your day. Flexibility in scheduling allows for adjustments when life gets busy, ensuring that exercise remains a priority.

With goals, preferences, and time constraints in mind, it's time to select the types of exercises that will form the core of your routine. A well-rounded fitness plan typically includes a mix of aerobic, strength, flexibility, and balance exercises. Aerobic activities, such as walking, cycling, or swimming, improve cardiovascular health and endurance. Strength training, using weights or bodyweight exercises, builds muscle and supports metabolic health. Flexibility exercises, like yoga or stretching, enhance mobility and prevent injury. Balance exercises, such as tai chi or simple balance drills, improve stability and coordination.

Creating a balanced routine involves determining the frequency, intensity, and duration of each type of exercise. For beginners, starting with moderate-intensity aerobic exercise for at least 150 minutes per week, combined with two to three strength training sessions, is a solid foundation. Flexibility and balance exercises can be incorporated into warm-ups or cool-downs, or practiced on rest days. As fitness levels improve, gradually increasing intensity and duration can help continue progress and prevent plateaus.

Listening to your body is paramount when designing and following an exercise routine. Pay attention to how your body responds to different activities and adjust accordingly. If an exercise causes pain or discomfort, modify it or try an alternative. Rest and recovery are equally important, allowing the body to repair and grow stronger. Incorporating rest days and varying the intensity of workouts can prevent overtraining and reduce the risk of injury.

Tracking progress is a valuable tool in maintaining motivation and assessing the effectiveness of your routine. Keep a journal or use a fitness app to record workouts, noting any improvements in strength, endurance, or flexibility. Celebrate milestones and achievements, no matter how small, as they signify progress and reinforce commitment to your goals.

As you become more comfortable with your routine, don't be afraid to experiment and make changes. Fitness is a dynamic journey, and what works today may need adjustment tomorrow. Trying new activities, increasing intensity, or setting new goals can keep the routine fresh and challenging. This adaptability ensures that your exercise plan evolves with you, supporting your growth and development.

Incorporating social elements into your exercise routine can enhance enjoyment and accountability. Joining a fitness class, participating in group sports, or finding a workout buddy can provide camaraderie and motivation. Sharing the experience with others can make exercise more enjoyable and foster a sense of community and support.

Nutrition and hydration are integral components of a successful exercise routine. Fueling your body with balanced meals and staying hydrated supports performance and recovery. Pay attention to pre- and post-workout nutrition, ensuring that you consume adequate carbohydrates, proteins, and fluids to sustain energy levels and promote muscle repair.

The Benefits of Strength Training

Strength training, often synonymous with lifting weights, is a powerful tool that extends far beyond the realm of bodybuilding. It offers a myriad of benefits that enhance physical health, mental well-being, and overall quality of life. Whether you're a seasoned athlete or a fitness novice, incorporating strength training into your routine can yield transformative results.

At its core, strength training involves exercises that improve muscle strength and endurance by working against resistance. This resistance can come from free weights, resistance bands, machines, or even your own body weight. The primary goal is to challenge the muscles, prompting them to adapt and grow stronger over time. This adaptation process is not only about building muscle mass but also about enhancing the body's functional capabilities.

One of the most significant benefits of strength training is its impact on muscle mass and metabolism. As we age, we naturally lose muscle mass, a process known as sarcopenia. This loss can lead to decreased strength, mobility, and independence. Strength training counteracts this decline by stimulating muscle growth and maintenance. Increased muscle mass also boosts resting metabolic rate, meaning you burn more calories even at rest. This can be particularly beneficial for weight management and fat loss.

Beyond muscle growth, strength training plays a crucial role in bone health. Weight-bearing exercises stimulate bone formation and increase bone density, reducing the risk of osteoporosis and fractures. This is especially important for postmenopausal women, who are at a higher risk of bone density loss. By incorporating regular strength training, individuals can fortify their skeletal system and maintain bone health well into their later years.

Strength training also enhances joint function and stability. By strengthening the muscles surrounding the joints, it provides better support and reduces the risk of injury. This is particularly beneficial for individuals with arthritis or joint pain, as stronger muscles can alleviate stress on the joints and improve mobility. Additionally, strength training can correct muscle imbalances and improve posture, further contributing to joint health and overall physical alignment.

The cardiovascular benefits of strength training are often overlooked, yet they are substantial. While it may not provide the same immediate cardiovascular workout as aerobic exercises, strength training contributes to heart health by improving circulation, lowering blood pressure, and reducing cholesterol levels. It also enhances insulin sensitivity, which can help prevent or manage type 2 diabetes. When combined with aerobic exercise, strength training creates a comprehensive fitness regimen that supports cardiovascular health.

Mental health is another area where strength training shines. Engaging in regular resistance exercises has been shown to reduce symptoms of anxiety and depression, boost mood, and enhance cognitive function. The act of lifting weights can be empowering, fostering a sense of accomplishment and boosting self-esteem. The focus and discipline required during strength training sessions can also serve as a form of mindfulness, providing a mental break from daily stressors.

Strength training is highly adaptable and can be tailored to suit individual needs and goals. Whether you're looking to build muscle, improve athletic performance, or simply enhance daily functioning, there are exercises and routines to match your objectives. Beginners can start with basic bodyweight exercises, such as squats, push-ups, and lunges, gradually progressing to more challenging movements and incorporating weights or resistance bands.

For those concerned about time constraints, strength training can be efficiently integrated into a busy schedule. Short, high-intensity sessions can be just as effective as longer workouts, provided they are performed with proper form and intensity. Circuit training, which involves performing a series of exercises with minimal rest in between, is an excellent way to maximize efficiency and keep workouts engaging.

Safety is paramount when engaging in strength training. Proper form and technique are essential to

prevent injury and ensure that exercises are effective.
It's advisable to start with lighter weights and focus on
mastering the movements before progressing to
heavier loads. Consulting with a certified trainer or
attending a strength training class can provide
valuable guidance and support, especially for
beginners.

Recovery is an integral part of any strength training
program. Muscles need time to repair and grow
stronger after being challenged, so incorporating rest
days and varying the intensity of workouts is crucial.
Adequate nutrition and hydration also play a vital role
in recovery, providing the necessary building blocks
for muscle repair and growth.

Strength training is not just for the young or athletic;
it is a lifelong practice that can benefit individuals of
all ages and fitness levels. Older adults, in particular,
can reap significant rewards from resistance exercises,
as they help maintain independence, mobility, and
quality of life. By embracing strength training,
individuals can empower themselves to lead healthier,
more active lives.

Flexibility and Balance Exercises

Flexibility and balance exercises are often the unsung
heroes of a well-rounded fitness regimen. While they
may not garner the same attention as high-intensity
workouts or strength training, their importance
cannot be overstated. These exercises play a crucial
role in maintaining mobility, preventing injury, and
enhancing overall physical performance. By
incorporating flexibility and balance work into your

routine, you can improve your body's functionality and resilience, paving the way for a healthier, more active lifestyle.

Flexibility exercises focus on lengthening muscles and increasing the range of motion in the joints. This is essential for maintaining mobility and preventing stiffness, particularly as we age. Stretching is the most common form of flexibility exercise, and it can be performed in various ways, including static, dynamic, and proprioceptive neuromuscular facilitation (PNF) stretching. Each method offers unique benefits and can be tailored to individual needs and preferences.

Static stretching involves holding a stretch for a period of time, typically 15 to 60 seconds, allowing the muscles to relax and lengthen. This type of stretching is ideal for improving flexibility and is often performed after a workout when the muscles are warm. Dynamic stretching, on the other hand, involves moving parts of the body through a full range of motion, gradually increasing reach and speed. This method is particularly effective as a warm-up, preparing the body for physical activity by increasing blood flow and reducing the risk of injury.

PNF stretching is a more advanced technique that combines passive stretching and isometric contractions. It is often used in rehabilitation settings to improve flexibility and range of motion. While it can be highly effective, it is recommended to perform PNF stretching under the guidance of a trained professional to ensure safety and effectiveness.

Incorporating flexibility exercises into your routine can be as simple as dedicating a few minutes to stretching each day. Focus on major muscle groups, such as the hamstrings, quadriceps, hip flexors, and shoulders, and hold each stretch gently without bouncing. Consistency is key, and over time, you will notice improvements in your flexibility and overall comfort in daily activities.

Balance exercises, while often overlooked, are equally important for maintaining stability and preventing falls. These exercises challenge the body's ability to maintain equilibrium, enhancing coordination and proprioception. Balance work is particularly beneficial for older adults, athletes, and individuals recovering from injury, as it strengthens the core and lower body muscles that support stability.

Simple balance exercises can be performed almost anywhere and require minimal equipment. Standing on one leg, walking heel-to-toe, or using a balance board are effective ways to challenge your balance. Tai chi, a gentle form of martial arts, is also an excellent practice for improving balance and coordination. Its slow, controlled movements promote mindfulness and relaxation, making it a holistic approach to balance training.

Yoga and Pilates are popular practices that combine flexibility and balance exercises, offering a comprehensive approach to fitness. Yoga focuses on postures, breathing, and meditation, enhancing flexibility, balance, and mental well-being. Pilates emphasizes core strength, alignment, and controlled movements, improving posture and stability. Both practices can be adapted to suit different fitness levels and provide a supportive environment for developing flexibility and balance.

Incorporating flexibility and balance exercises into your fitness routine offers numerous benefits beyond physical health. These exercises promote relaxation and stress relief, contributing to mental and emotional well-being. The focus and concentration required during balance exercises can serve as a form of mindfulness, providing a mental break from daily stressors. Flexibility work, particularly when combined with deep breathing, can release tension and promote a sense of calm and relaxation.

To maximize the benefits of flexibility and balance exercises, it's important to approach them with patience and consistency. Progress may be gradual, but with regular practice, you will notice improvements in your range of motion, stability, and overall physical performance. Listening to your body and respecting its limits is crucial, as pushing too hard can lead to injury. Instead, focus on gradual progress and celebrate small achievements along the way.

Flexibility and balance exercises are not just for athletes or fitness enthusiasts; they are essential components of a healthy lifestyle for individuals of all ages and fitness levels. By incorporating these exercises into your routine, you can enhance your body's functionality, prevent injury, and improve your quality of life. Whether you're stretching in the morning, practicing yoga in the evening, or performing balance drills during a break, these exercises offer a pathway to a more balanced and flexible life.

Staying Motivated and Consistent

Motivation and consistency are the twin pillars of any successful fitness journey. While the initial excitement of starting a new exercise routine can be invigorating, maintaining that enthusiasm over the long haul often proves challenging. Life's demands, unexpected obstacles, and even the monotony of routine can sap motivation, making it difficult to stay on track. However, by understanding the dynamics of motivation and employing strategies to foster consistency, you can cultivate a sustainable fitness lifestyle that endures beyond fleeting bursts of inspiration.

The first step in staying motivated is to establish a clear and compelling "why." This involves identifying the deeper reasons behind your fitness goals. Are you seeking to improve your health, boost your energy levels, or enhance your self-confidence? Perhaps you want to set a positive example for your family or prepare for an upcoming event. Whatever your reasons, having a strong and personal motivation can serve as a powerful anchor when challenges arise. Write down your "why" and revisit it regularly to remind yourself of the purpose behind your efforts.

Setting specific, measurable, achievable, relevant, and time-bound (SMART) goals is another effective way to maintain motivation. Instead of vague aspirations like "get fit," define clear objectives such as "run a 5K in three months" or "attend yoga class twice a week." These goals provide direction and allow you to track progress, which can be incredibly motivating. Celebrate small victories along the way, as they signify progress and reinforce your commitment to your goals.

Creating a structured routine is essential for building consistency. Designate specific times for exercise and treat them as non-negotiable appointments with yourself. Consistency in scheduling helps establish a habit, making it easier to stick to your routine even when motivation wanes. Consider your daily schedule and identify windows of time that are most conducive to exercise, whether it's early in the morning, during lunch breaks, or in the evening. By prioritizing these sessions, you reinforce the importance of fitness in your life.

Variety is the spice of life, and it plays a crucial role in maintaining motivation. Engaging in the same workout day after day can lead to boredom and burnout. To keep things fresh and exciting, incorporate a mix of activities into your routine. Try new classes, explore different outdoor activities, or experiment with various workout formats. This not only prevents monotony but also challenges your body in new ways, promoting overall fitness and preventing plateaus.

Accountability is a powerful motivator. Sharing your fitness goals with a friend, family member, or workout partner can provide the support and encouragement needed to stay on track. Consider joining a fitness group or class where you can connect with like-minded individuals who share similar goals. The camaraderie and shared experiences can foster a sense of community and make exercise more enjoyable. Additionally, tracking your progress through a journal or fitness app can hold you accountable and provide tangible evidence of your achievements.

It's important to recognize that motivation naturally fluctuates. There will be days when you feel energized and eager to exercise, and others when the couch seems far more appealing. On those challenging days, focus on the discipline of showing up rather than the intensity of the workout. Even a short, low-intensity session can reinforce the habit and keep you moving forward. Remember that consistency is built on the accumulation of small, consistent actions over time.

Listening to your body is crucial in maintaining both motivation and consistency. Pay attention to how your body feels and adjust your routine accordingly. If you're feeling fatigued or experiencing discomfort, allow yourself to rest and recover. Overtraining can lead to burnout and injury, derailing your progress. By honoring your body's needs, you create a sustainable approach to fitness that supports long-term success.

Mindset plays a significant role in staying motivated. Cultivate a positive and growth-oriented mindset by focusing on progress rather than perfection. Embrace setbacks as opportunities to learn and grow, rather than as failures. Celebrate your efforts and achievements, no matter how small, and practice self-compassion on days when things don't go as planned. By fostering a mindset of resilience and adaptability, you empower yourself to navigate the ups and downs of your fitness journey.

Incorporating elements of fun and enjoyment into your routine can also enhance motivation. Choose activities that you genuinely enjoy and look forward to, whether it's dancing, hiking, or playing a sport. Exercise doesn't have to be a chore; it can be a source of joy and fulfillment. By aligning your fitness routine with your interests and passions, you create a positive association with exercise that fuels motivation.

Finally, remember that motivation is not a finite resource; it can be cultivated and replenished. Regularly revisit your goals, reflect on your progress, and adjust your routine as needed to keep things fresh and aligned with your evolving aspirations. Surround yourself with positive influences, whether it's inspiring books, podcasts, or role models who embody the values you aspire to. By nurturing your motivation and committing to consistency, you lay the foundation for a lifelong journey of health and well-being.

Chapter 4

Mind-Body Connection

The Role of Mental Health in Physical Wellness

The intricate connection between mental health and physical wellness is a dynamic interplay that significantly influences overall well-being. While physical fitness often takes center stage in discussions about health, the role of mental health is equally crucial. Understanding this relationship can empower individuals to adopt a holistic approach to wellness, where both mind and body are nurtured and supported.

Mental health encompasses emotional, psychological, and social well-being, affecting how we think, feel, and act. It influences our ability to handle stress, relate to others, and make choices. When mental health is compromised, it can manifest in various ways, impacting physical health and daily functioning. Conversely, a strong mental state can enhance physical performance, resilience, and recovery.

Stress is a common factor that bridges the gap between mental and physical health. Chronic stress can lead to a cascade of physiological responses, including increased heart rate, elevated blood pressure, and the release of stress hormones like cortisol. Over time, these responses can contribute to the development of chronic conditions such as heart disease, obesity, and diabetes. Stress can also weaken the immune system, making the body more susceptible to infections and illnesses.

Exercise is a powerful tool for managing stress and improving mental health. Physical activity stimulates the production of endorphins, the body's natural mood elevators, which can alleviate feelings of anxiety and depression. Regular exercise also promotes better sleep, which is essential for mental and physical recovery. By incorporating physical activity into daily life, individuals can create a positive feedback loop that enhances both mental and physical health.

Mindfulness and meditation are practices that can further support mental health and, by extension, physical wellness. These practices encourage individuals to focus on the present moment, reducing stress and promoting relaxation. Mindfulness has been shown to lower blood pressure, improve immune function, and enhance overall well-being. By integrating mindfulness into a fitness routine, individuals can cultivate a sense of balance and harmony between mind and body.

Social connections play a vital role in mental health and can influence physical wellness. Strong social support networks provide emotional comfort, reduce stress, and promote a sense of belonging. Engaging in group activities, such as fitness classes or team sports, can foster social connections and enhance motivation. These interactions not only boost mental health but also encourage adherence to physical activity, contributing to overall wellness.

Nutrition is another critical component that links mental health and physical wellness. A balanced diet rich in nutrients supports brain function and emotional stability. Certain nutrients, such as omega-3 fatty acids, B vitamins, and antioxidants, have been shown to improve mood and cognitive function. Conversely, a diet high in processed foods and sugar can negatively impact mental health, leading to mood swings and fatigue. By prioritizing a nutritious diet, individuals can support both mental clarity and physical vitality.

Sleep is a fundamental aspect of mental health that directly affects physical wellness. Quality sleep is essential for cognitive function, emotional regulation, and physical recovery. Sleep deprivation can lead to irritability, impaired decision-making, and decreased physical performance. Establishing a consistent sleep routine and creating a restful environment can enhance sleep quality, supporting overall health and well-being.

The mind-body connection is further exemplified in the practice of yoga, which combines physical postures, breathing exercises, and meditation. Yoga promotes flexibility, strength, and balance while also fostering mental clarity and relaxation. This holistic approach to wellness highlights the interconnectedness of mental and physical health, offering a pathway to greater harmony and balance.

It's important to recognize that mental health challenges can affect anyone, regardless of age or fitness level. Seeking support from mental health professionals, such as therapists or counselors, can provide valuable guidance and coping strategies. Therapy can help individuals address underlying issues, develop resilience, and improve their overall quality of life.

Incorporating mental health practices into a wellness routine requires intention and commitment. Start by setting aside time each day for activities that promote relaxation and self-care, whether it's meditation, journaling, or spending time in nature. These practices can help reduce stress, enhance mood, and improve overall well-being.

Building a strong foundation of mental health can enhance physical wellness and vice versa. By nurturing both aspects of health, individuals can achieve a more balanced and fulfilling life. Embrace the journey of holistic wellness, where the mind and body work in harmony to support your overall health and happiness.

Stress Management Techniques

Stress is an inevitable part of life, a natural response to the challenges and demands we face daily. While a certain level of stress can be motivating, chronic stress can have detrimental effects on both mental and physical health. It can lead to anxiety, depression, sleep disturbances, and a host of physical ailments, including heart disease and weakened immunity. Therefore, mastering stress management techniques is essential for maintaining overall well-being and enhancing quality of life.

One of the most effective ways to manage stress is through mindfulness meditation. This practice involves focusing on the present moment, acknowledging thoughts and feelings without judgment. By cultivating awareness and acceptance, mindfulness meditation can reduce stress and promote relaxation. It encourages a shift in perspective, allowing individuals to respond to stressors with greater clarity and calmness. Setting aside just a few minutes each day for mindfulness meditation can create a profound impact, fostering a sense of peace and balance.

Deep breathing exercises are another powerful tool for stress management. When stress strikes, the body's natural response is to enter a state of heightened alertness, often accompanied by shallow, rapid breathing. Deep breathing techniques counteract this response by activating the parasympathetic nervous system, which promotes relaxation. Practicing deep, slow breaths can lower heart rate, reduce blood pressure, and induce a state of calm. Techniques such as diaphragmatic breathing, where you focus on expanding the diaphragm rather than the chest, can be practiced anywhere and anytime stress arises.

Physical activity is a well-documented stress reliever. Exercise releases endorphins, the body's natural mood enhancers, which can alleviate stress and improve mood. Whether it's a brisk walk, a yoga session, or a high-intensity workout, physical activity provides an outlet for releasing tension and pent-up energy. Regular exercise also improves sleep quality, boosts self-esteem, and enhances overall resilience to stress. Finding an activity you enjoy and incorporating it into your routine can be a powerful strategy for managing stress.

Progressive muscle relaxation is a technique that involves systematically tensing and then relaxing different muscle groups in the body. This practice helps individuals become more aware of physical sensations associated with stress and tension, promoting relaxation and reducing stress. By focusing on the contrast between tension and relaxation, individuals can learn to release physical stress and achieve a state of calm. Progressive muscle relaxation can be particularly beneficial before bedtime, aiding in restful sleep.

Time management is a practical approach to reducing stress. Feeling overwhelmed by a long to-do list or looming deadlines can exacerbate stress levels. By prioritizing tasks, setting realistic goals, and breaking projects into manageable steps, individuals can regain a sense of control and reduce stress. Techniques such as creating a daily schedule, setting boundaries, and delegating tasks can help manage time effectively and prevent burnout.

Social support is a crucial element in stress management. Connecting with friends, family, or support groups provides emotional comfort and a sense of belonging. Sharing experiences and feelings with others can alleviate stress and provide new perspectives on challenges. Building a strong support network and reaching out for help when needed can enhance resilience and provide a buffer against stress.

Journaling is a therapeutic practice that allows individuals to express thoughts and emotions, gaining insight into stressors and triggers. Writing about stressful experiences can help process emotions, identify patterns, and develop coping strategies.

Journaling provides a safe space for self-reflection and can be a valuable tool for managing stress and promoting emotional well-being.

Laughter is often referred to as the best medicine, and for good reason. Laughter triggers the release of endorphins, reduces stress hormones, and increases immune function. Engaging in activities that bring joy and laughter, whether it's watching a comedy, spending time with loved ones, or participating in a fun hobby, can significantly reduce stress and enhance mood.

A healthy diet plays a vital role in stress management. Nutrient-rich foods support brain function and emotional stability, while a diet high in processed foods and sugar can exacerbate stress and mood swings. Incorporating foods rich in omega-3 fatty acids, antioxidants, and vitamins can support mental health and resilience to stress. Staying hydrated and avoiding excessive caffeine and alcohol intake can also help maintain balance and reduce stress.

Sleep is a cornerstone of stress management. Quality sleep is essential for cognitive function, emotional regulation, and physical recovery. Sleep deprivation can increase stress levels and impair decision-making. Establishing a consistent sleep routine, creating a restful environment, and practicing relaxation techniques before bedtime can enhance sleep quality and support overall well-being.

Incorporating stress management techniques into daily life requires intention and practice. Start by identifying the techniques that resonate most with you and gradually integrate them into your routine.

Consistency is key, and over time, these practices can become second nature, providing a foundation for resilience and well-being.

Mindfulness and Meditation Practices

Mindfulness and meditation have emerged as powerful practices for cultivating mental clarity, emotional balance, and overall well-being. In a world that often feels chaotic and fast-paced, these practices offer a refuge—a way to anchor oneself in the present moment and find peace amidst the noise. By integrating mindfulness and meditation into daily life, individuals can enhance their mental and physical health, improve focus, and foster a deeper connection with themselves and the world around them.

Mindfulness is the practice of paying attention to the present moment with openness, curiosity, and without judgment. It involves being fully aware of your thoughts, emotions, and sensations as they arise, allowing you to experience life more vividly and authentically. Mindfulness can be practiced in various ways, from formal meditation sessions to informal moments of awareness throughout the day.

One of the simplest ways to practice mindfulness is through mindful breathing. This involves focusing your attention on the natural rhythm of your breath, observing each inhale and exhale without trying to change it. As thoughts inevitably arise, acknowledge them without judgment and gently return your focus to the breath. This practice can be done anywhere, whether you're sitting quietly at home or taking a moment to pause during a busy day. Mindful breathing helps calm the mind, reduce stress, and bring a sense of grounding and presence.

Body scan meditation is another effective mindfulness practice. It involves systematically bringing attention to different parts of the body, noticing any sensations, tension, or discomfort. Starting from the toes and working your way up to the head, the body scan encourages relaxation and awareness of physical sensations. This practice can help release tension, improve body awareness, and promote a sense of relaxation and well-being.

Mindful walking is a practice that combines movement with mindfulness. As you walk, focus on the sensations of each step—the feeling of your feet touching the ground, the movement of your legs, and the rhythm of your breath. Walking mindfully allows you to connect with your surroundings and experience the present moment fully. It's a wonderful way to incorporate mindfulness into daily life, whether you're walking in nature or simply moving from one place to another.

Meditation, while often associated with mindfulness, encompasses a broader range of practices aimed at cultivating mental clarity and inner peace. There are various forms of meditation, each with its unique focus and techniques. One popular form is loving-kindness meditation, which involves directing positive intentions and well-wishes toward yourself and others. This practice fosters compassion, empathy, and a sense of interconnectedness with others.

Another form of meditation is focused attention meditation, where you concentrate on a single point of focus, such as a mantra, a candle flame, or the breath. This practice helps develop concentration and mental discipline, allowing you to quiet the mind and experience a sense of inner stillness. Over time, focused attention meditation can enhance cognitive function, improve attention span, and reduce stress.

Open awareness meditation, also known as choiceless awareness, involves observing thoughts, emotions, and sensations as they arise without attachment or judgment. This practice encourages a state of relaxed awareness, where you become an impartial witness to your inner experience. Open awareness meditation can lead to greater self-awareness, emotional regulation, and a deeper understanding of the mind's nature.

Incorporating mindfulness and meditation into daily life requires intention and commitment. Start by setting aside a few minutes each day for practice, gradually increasing the duration as you become more comfortable. Consistency is key, and over time, these practices can become a natural and integral part of your routine.

Creating a dedicated space for meditation can enhance your practice. Choose a quiet, comfortable area where you can sit or lie down without distractions. Consider adding elements that promote relaxation, such as cushions, candles, or calming music. Having a designated space can signal to your mind and body that it's time to relax and focus inward.

It's important to approach mindfulness and meditation with an open mind and a sense of curiosity. There is no right or wrong way to practice, and each session may bring different experiences and insights. Be patient with yourself and embrace the journey of self-discovery and growth.

The benefits of mindfulness and meditation extend beyond the individual, influencing relationships and interactions with others. By cultivating a sense of presence and empathy, these practices can enhance communication, deepen connections, and foster a sense of compassion and understanding. As you become more attuned to your own thoughts and emotions, you may find it easier to navigate conflicts and respond to others with kindness and patience.

Mindfulness and meditation also have a profound impact on physical health. Research has shown that these practices can reduce stress, lower blood pressure, improve immune function, and enhance overall well-being. By promoting relaxation and reducing the physiological effects of stress, mindfulness and meditation support the body's natural healing processes and contribute to a healthier, more balanced life.

Incorporating mindfulness and meditation into your daily routine can transform your relationship with yourself and the world around you. These practices offer a pathway to greater self-awareness, emotional resilience, and inner peace. By embracing mindfulness and meditation, you can cultivate a state of presence and clarity that enriches every aspect of your life.

The Impact of Sleep on Well-Being

Sleep is a fundamental pillar of well-being, intricately linked to both physical health and mental clarity. Despite its importance, sleep is often undervalued in our fast-paced society, where the demands of work, family, and social obligations can encroach upon the time needed for restorative rest. Understanding the profound impact of sleep on well-being can inspire individuals to prioritize this essential aspect of health, leading to improved quality of life and enhanced overall functioning.

The human body operates on a circadian rhythm, a natural internal clock that regulates the sleep-wake cycle over a 24-hour period. This rhythm is influenced by external cues such as light and temperature, which signal the body when to feel alert and when to wind down. Disruptions to this rhythm, whether due to irregular sleep schedules, shift work, or excessive screen time, can lead to sleep disturbances and a cascade of negative effects on health.

Quality sleep is crucial for cognitive function, affecting memory, attention, and problem-solving abilities. During sleep, the brain consolidates memories, processes information, and clears out toxins that accumulate during waking hours. A lack of sleep can impair these processes, leading to forgetfulness, difficulty concentrating, and decreased productivity. For students and professionals alike, prioritizing sleep can enhance learning and performance, providing a competitive edge in academic and work environments.

Emotional regulation is another area profoundly influenced by sleep. Insufficient sleep can heighten emotional reactivity, making individuals more prone to mood swings, irritability, and stress. Chronic sleep deprivation has been linked to an increased risk of developing mood disorders such as anxiety and depression. By ensuring adequate rest, individuals can bolster their emotional resilience, better managing stress and maintaining a positive outlook on life.

Physical health is deeply intertwined with sleep quality. During deep sleep stages, the body undergoes critical repair and regeneration processes, including muscle growth, tissue repair, and the release of growth hormones. Sleep also plays a vital role in immune function, with studies showing that well-rested individuals are better equipped to fend off infections and illnesses. Conversely, chronic sleep deprivation can weaken the immune system, increasing susceptibility to colds, flu, and other ailments.

Metabolic health is another area where sleep exerts significant influence. Sleep deprivation can disrupt the balance of hormones that regulate appetite, leading to increased hunger and cravings for high-calorie foods. This can contribute to weight gain and increase the risk of obesity and related conditions such as type 2 diabetes. By prioritizing sleep, individuals can support healthy metabolism and weight management, reducing the risk of chronic diseases.

The relationship between sleep and cardiovascular health is well-documented. Poor sleep quality and short sleep duration have been associated with an increased risk of hypertension, heart disease, and stroke. Sleep helps regulate blood pressure and supports heart health by reducing inflammation and stress on the cardiovascular system. Ensuring sufficient sleep can be a protective factor against heart-related conditions, promoting longevity and vitality.

Creating a sleep-friendly environment is essential for optimizing rest. This involves minimizing noise and light disruptions, maintaining a comfortable room temperature, and investing in a supportive mattress and pillows. Establishing a consistent sleep schedule, where you go to bed and wake up at the same time each day, can reinforce the body's natural circadian rhythm and improve sleep quality.

Limiting exposure to screens and electronic devices before bedtime is crucial, as the blue light emitted by screens can interfere with the production of melatonin, the hormone that regulates sleep. Instead, consider engaging in relaxing activities such as reading, taking a warm bath, or practicing gentle yoga or meditation to signal to your body that it's time to wind down.

Diet and lifestyle choices also play a role in sleep quality. Consuming caffeine or heavy meals close to bedtime can disrupt sleep, while regular physical activity can promote deeper, more restful sleep. However, it's important to avoid vigorous exercise too close to bedtime, as it can have a stimulating effect. Finding a balance that works for your body can enhance sleep and overall well-being.

For those who struggle with sleep disturbances, such as insomnia or sleep apnea, seeking professional help is important. Sleep specialists can provide guidance and treatment options to address underlying issues and improve sleep quality. Cognitive-behavioral therapy for insomnia (CBT-I) is an evidence-based approach that can help individuals develop healthier sleep habits and overcome sleep-related challenges.

Incorporating mindfulness and relaxation techniques into your bedtime routine can also support better sleep. Practices such as deep breathing, progressive muscle relaxation, and guided imagery can calm the mind and prepare the body for rest. By creating a sense of tranquility and letting go of the day's stresses, these techniques can facilitate a smoother transition into sleep.

The impact of sleep on well-being is profound and far-reaching, influencing every aspect of health and daily functioning. By prioritizing sleep and adopting habits that support restorative rest, individuals can enhance their cognitive, emotional, and physical health. Embracing the power of sleep as a cornerstone of well-being can lead to a more balanced, vibrant, and fulfilling life.

Cultivating Positive Relationships

Positive relationships are the cornerstone of a fulfilling and meaningful life. They provide emotional support, foster a sense of belonging, and contribute to overall well-being. Cultivating these relationships requires intention, effort, and a willingness to invest in the connections that matter most. By nurturing positive relationships, individuals can enhance their happiness, resilience, and personal growth.

At the heart of positive relationships lies effective communication. Open, honest, and empathetic communication is essential for building trust and understanding. It involves not only expressing your thoughts and feelings but also actively listening to others. Listening with empathy means being fully present, acknowledging the other person's perspective, and responding with compassion. This creates a safe space for open dialogue, where both parties feel heard and valued.

Empathy is a powerful tool for deepening relationships. It involves putting yourself in someone else's shoes and understanding their emotions and experiences. By practicing empathy, you can strengthen your connections and foster a sense of mutual respect and understanding. Empathy can be cultivated through active listening, asking open-ended questions, and being genuinely curious about the other person's experiences.

Shared experiences and activities are another way to cultivate positive relationships. Engaging in activities that both parties enjoy can create lasting memories and strengthen bonds. Whether it's cooking a meal together, going for a hike, or attending a concert, shared experiences provide opportunities for connection and joy. These activities can also serve as a foundation for building trust and intimacy, as they allow individuals to learn more about each other's interests and values.

Setting healthy boundaries is crucial for maintaining positive relationships. Boundaries define what is acceptable and unacceptable behavior, ensuring that both parties feel respected and valued. Communicating boundaries clearly and assertively can prevent misunderstandings and conflicts. It's important to remember that boundaries are not about creating distance but about fostering a healthy and balanced relationship where both parties feel comfortable and respected.

Conflict is a natural part of any relationship, but how it is handled can make all the difference. Approaching conflicts with a mindset of collaboration and problem-solving can lead to positive outcomes. This involves focusing on the issue at hand, avoiding blame, and seeking solutions that benefit both parties. By addressing conflicts constructively, individuals can strengthen their relationships and build a foundation of trust and respect.

Gratitude is a powerful practice for enhancing relationships. Expressing appreciation for the people in your life can strengthen bonds and foster a sense of connection. Whether it's a simple thank you, a heartfelt note, or a small gesture of kindness, showing gratitude can make others feel valued and appreciated. Practicing gratitude also shifts your focus to the positive aspects of your relationships, enhancing your overall sense of well-being.

Vulnerability is an essential component of deep and meaningful relationships. It involves being open and honest about your thoughts, feelings, and experiences, even when it feels uncomfortable. By embracing vulnerability, you create an environment of trust and authenticity, where both parties feel safe to be themselves. Vulnerability can lead to deeper connections and a greater sense of intimacy, as it allows individuals to share their true selves without fear of judgment.

Investing time and energy into relationships is key to their growth and sustainability. Regularly checking in with loved ones, making time for meaningful conversations, and being present in their lives can strengthen connections and foster a sense of closeness. It's important to prioritize relationships and make them a central part of your life, as they provide support, joy, and a sense of belonging.

Diversity and inclusivity are important considerations in cultivating positive relationships. Embracing diversity means valuing and respecting differences in culture, background, and perspective. By fostering an inclusive environment, you create a space where everyone feels welcome and valued. This can lead to richer and more meaningful relationships, as it allows individuals to learn from each other's unique experiences and viewpoints.

Self-awareness is a critical aspect of building positive relationships. Understanding your own emotions, triggers, and communication style can help you navigate interactions more effectively. By being aware of your strengths and areas for growth, you can approach relationships with greater empathy and understanding. Self-awareness also allows you to take responsibility for your actions and make positive changes that enhance your relationships.

Forgiveness is a powerful practice for healing and strengthening relationships. Holding onto grudges and resentment can create distance and tension, while forgiveness allows for healing and reconciliation. Forgiveness involves letting go of past hurts and focusing on the present and future. It doesn't mean condoning harmful behavior, but rather releasing the emotional burden and choosing to move forward with compassion and understanding.

Chapter 5
Creating a Healthy Lifestyle

Building Healthy Habits

Building healthy habits is a transformative journey that can lead to lasting improvements in physical health, mental well-being, and overall quality of life. Habits are the small decisions and actions we make every day, and they shape our lives in profound ways. By consciously cultivating positive habits, individuals can create a foundation for success and fulfillment.

The process of building healthy habits begins with self-awareness and intention. Understanding your current habits and identifying areas for improvement is the first step. Take a moment to reflect on your daily routines and behaviors. Are there habits that no longer serve you or align with your goals? Are there new habits you wish to cultivate? By gaining clarity on your intentions, you can set a clear path for change.

Setting specific, achievable goals is crucial for habit formation. Vague intentions often lead to inconsistent efforts, while clear goals provide direction and motivation. Instead of setting a broad goal like "get healthier," break it down into specific actions, such as "exercise for 30 minutes three times a week" or "eat a serving of vegetables with every meal." These concrete goals are easier to track and achieve, providing a sense of accomplishment and momentum.

Consistency is the cornerstone of habit formation. Repetition reinforces behavior, gradually turning actions into automatic responses. Start small and focus on one habit at a time, allowing yourself to build confidence and establish a routine. For example, if your goal is to incorporate meditation into your daily life, begin with just five minutes a day and gradually increase the duration as it becomes a natural part of your routine.

Creating an environment that supports your goals can significantly impact your success. Surround yourself with cues and reminders that encourage positive behavior. If you're aiming to eat healthier, stock your kitchen with nutritious foods and keep tempting snacks out of sight. If you want to exercise regularly, lay out your workout clothes the night before or schedule workouts with a friend for accountability. By designing your environment to align with your goals, you reduce friction and make it easier to stick to your habits.

Tracking your progress is a powerful motivator. Keeping a journal or using a habit-tracking app can help you monitor your efforts and celebrate your achievements. Seeing tangible evidence of your progress reinforces your commitment and provides a sense of accomplishment. It also allows you to identify patterns and make adjustments as needed, ensuring that your habits continue to align with your goals.

Overcoming obstacles is an inevitable part of building healthy habits. Life is unpredictable, and setbacks are bound to occur. The key is to approach challenges with resilience and adaptability. Instead of viewing setbacks as failures, see them as opportunities to learn and grow. Reflect on what went wrong, adjust your approach, and recommit to your goals. Remember that progress is not always linear, and every step forward, no matter how small, is a step in the right direction.

Mindfulness can play a significant role in habit formation. By cultivating awareness of your thoughts, emotions, and behaviors, you can make conscious choices that align with your goals. Mindfulness helps you recognize triggers and automatic responses, allowing you to interrupt negative patterns and replace them with positive actions. Practicing mindfulness can also enhance your ability to stay present and focused, reducing the likelihood of mindless habits that detract from your well-being.

Social support is a valuable asset in building healthy habits. Sharing your goals with friends, family, or a support group can provide encouragement, accountability, and motivation. Surrounding yourself with like-minded individuals who share similar goals can create a sense of community and camaraderie. Whether it's joining a fitness class, participating in a cooking club, or engaging in online forums, connecting with others can enhance your commitment and enjoyment of the journey.

Celebrating milestones and rewarding yourself for your efforts can reinforce positive behavior. Acknowledging your achievements, no matter how small, boosts motivation and self-esteem. Consider treating yourself to a relaxing activity, a new book, or a special outing as a reward for reaching a goal. These rewards serve as positive reinforcement, encouraging you to continue your efforts and maintain your habits.

Flexibility is an important aspect of sustaining healthy habits. Life is dynamic, and circumstances change. Be open to adjusting your goals and routines as needed to accommodate new challenges and opportunities. Flexibility allows you to adapt to life's demands while staying true to your intentions. By maintaining a growth mindset and embracing change, you can navigate obstacles with grace and resilience.

Building healthy habits is a lifelong journey, not a destination. It's about making intentional choices that align with your values and aspirations. By focusing on progress rather than perfection, you can cultivate a sense of fulfillment and well-being. Embrace the process, celebrate your successes, and learn from your experiences. With dedication and perseverance, you can create a life enriched by positive habits that support your health, happiness, and personal growth.

Time Management for Wellness

Time management is a crucial skill that directly impacts wellness, influencing both mental and physical health. In a world where demands on our time are ever-increasing, mastering the art of managing time effectively can lead to a more balanced and fulfilling life. By prioritizing tasks, setting boundaries, and making intentional choices, individuals can create space for activities that nurture their well-being.

The foundation of effective time management lies in understanding your priorities. Begin by identifying what truly matters to you, both personally and professionally. This involves reflecting on your values, goals, and aspirations. What activities bring you joy and fulfillment? What tasks are essential for your career or personal growth? By gaining clarity on your priorities, you can allocate your time and energy to the things that align with your values and contribute to your overall wellness.

Once you've identified your priorities, it's important to set clear and achievable goals. Break down larger goals into smaller, manageable tasks that can be accomplished within a specific timeframe. This approach not only makes goals more attainable but also provides a sense of progress and accomplishment. For example, if your goal is to improve your physical fitness, start by setting a target of exercising for 30 minutes three times a week. As you achieve these smaller milestones, you can gradually increase the intensity and frequency of your workouts.

Creating a structured schedule is a powerful tool for managing time effectively. Use a planner or digital calendar to organize your tasks and commitments. Allocate specific time slots for work, leisure, exercise, and self-care activities. By scheduling these activities, you ensure that they become a regular part of your routine, reducing the likelihood of neglecting important aspects of your wellness. Remember to include buffer time between tasks to accommodate unexpected events and prevent burnout.

Setting boundaries is essential for protecting your time and energy. Learn to say no to commitments that do not align with your priorities or that may overwhelm you. It's important to recognize that your time is valuable and that you have the right to protect it. Communicate your boundaries clearly and assertively, whether it's declining a social invitation or setting limits on work-related tasks. By setting boundaries, you create space for activities that support your well-being and prevent overcommitment.

Minimizing distractions is another key aspect of effective time management. Identify common distractions in your environment and take steps to reduce or eliminate them. This may involve turning off notifications on your phone, creating a dedicated workspace, or setting specific times to check emails and social media. By minimizing distractions, you can maintain focus and productivity, allowing you to complete tasks more efficiently and freeing up time for activities that enhance your wellness.

Incorporating mindfulness into your daily routine can enhance your time management skills. Mindfulness involves being fully present and engaged in the task at hand, reducing the tendency to multitask or become overwhelmed by competing demands. By practicing mindfulness, you can improve your concentration, make more intentional choices, and manage your time with greater awareness. Consider incorporating mindfulness practices such as meditation, deep breathing, or mindful walking into your day to enhance your focus and clarity.

Delegating tasks is an effective strategy for managing time and reducing stress. Recognize that you don't have to do everything yourself and that seeking help is a sign of strength, not weakness. Whether it's delegating tasks at work or sharing household responsibilities with family members, delegating allows you to focus on activities that align with your priorities and contribute to your wellness. Trust in the abilities of others and communicate your expectations clearly to ensure successful delegation.

Taking regular breaks is essential for maintaining productivity and preventing burnout. Schedule short breaks throughout your day to rest and recharge. Use this time to stretch, take a walk, or engage in a relaxing activity. Breaks provide an opportunity to clear your mind, reduce stress, and return to tasks with renewed focus and energy. Remember that taking breaks is not a sign of laziness but a necessary component of effective time management and overall wellness.

Reflecting on your time management practices is important for continuous improvement. At the end of each day or week, take a moment to review how you spent your time. Did you allocate your time in a way that aligns with your priorities? Were there any tasks or activities that could have been managed more effectively? Use this reflection as an opportunity to make adjustments and refine your time management strategies. By regularly evaluating your practices, you can identify areas for growth and make positive changes that enhance your wellness.

Incorporating self-care into your time management plan is crucial for maintaining balance and well-being. Self-care activities, such as exercise, relaxation, and hobbies, are essential for recharging your mind and body. Schedule regular self-care activities into your routine and treat them as non-negotiable commitments. By prioritizing self-care, you ensure that you have the energy and resilience to meet the demands of daily life and maintain your overall wellness.

Time management is a dynamic and ongoing process that requires flexibility and adaptability. Life is unpredictable, and circumstances can change unexpectedly. Be open to adjusting your plans and routines as needed to accommodate new challenges and opportunities. By maintaining a flexible mindset, you can navigate changes with ease and continue to prioritize your wellness.

The Importance of Routine

Routine serves as the backbone of daily life, providing structure and stability in an ever-changing world. It is the framework upon which we build our days, guiding us through the myriad tasks and responsibilities that demand our attention. The importance of routine extends beyond mere organization; it plays a crucial role in enhancing productivity, reducing stress, and promoting overall well-being.

Establishing a routine begins with understanding the rhythm of your day. Each person has a unique set of responsibilities, preferences, and energy levels that influence how they navigate their time. By observing your natural patterns, you can identify the optimal times for various activities, whether it's work, exercise, or relaxation. This self-awareness allows you to design a routine that aligns with your personal needs and maximizes your efficiency.

One of the primary benefits of routine is its ability to enhance productivity. When tasks are performed at consistent times, they become ingrained habits, requiring less mental effort and decision-making. This frees up cognitive resources for more complex tasks, allowing you to focus on what truly matters. For instance, setting aside a specific time each morning for planning and prioritizing can streamline your workflow and ensure that important tasks are addressed promptly.

Routine also provides a sense of predictability and control, which can significantly reduce stress and anxiety. In a world filled with uncertainties, having a reliable structure to your day can offer comfort and stability. Knowing what to expect and when to expect it allows you to approach each day with confidence, minimizing the mental strain of constant decision-making. This sense of control can be particularly beneficial during challenging times, providing a steady anchor amidst chaos.

Incorporating self-care into your routine is essential for maintaining balance and well-being. Self-care activities, such as exercise, meditation, or hobbies, should be treated as non-negotiable components of your day. By scheduling regular self-care practices, you prioritize your physical and mental health, ensuring that you have the energy and resilience to meet the demands of daily life. Whether it's a morning yoga session or an evening walk, these moments of self-care can rejuvenate your mind and body, enhancing your overall quality of life.

Routine can also foster a sense of accomplishment and motivation. Completing tasks and adhering to a schedule provides a tangible sense of progress, boosting self-esteem and encouraging further action.

This positive feedback loop reinforces the value of routine, motivating you to maintain and refine your daily structure. Celebrating small victories, such as completing a workout or finishing a project, can further enhance this sense of achievement and drive.

Flexibility within a routine is crucial for adapting to life's unpredictability. While structure is important, it's equally essential to remain open to change and adjust your routine as needed. Life is dynamic, and circumstances can shift unexpectedly. By maintaining a flexible mindset, you can navigate changes with ease, ensuring that your routine continues to serve your needs. This adaptability allows you to embrace new opportunities and challenges without feeling overwhelmed or constrained.

The social aspect of routine should not be overlooked. Regularly scheduled interactions with friends, family, or colleagues can strengthen relationships and foster a sense of community. Whether it's a weekly dinner with loved ones or a monthly book club meeting, these social routines provide opportunities for connection and support. By prioritizing social interactions, you nurture your emotional well-being and create a network of support that enriches your life.

Routine can also play a significant role in achieving long-term goals. By breaking down larger objectives into smaller, manageable tasks and incorporating them into your daily routine, you create a clear path toward success. This approach not only makes goals more attainable but also provides a sense of direction and purpose. For example, if your goal is to learn a new language, dedicating a specific time each day to practice can lead to steady progress and eventual mastery.

Incorporating mindfulness into your routine can enhance your overall well-being. Mindfulness involves being fully present and engaged in the moment, reducing the tendency to rush through tasks or become overwhelmed by competing demands. By practicing mindfulness, you can improve your concentration, make more intentional choices, and manage your time with greater awareness. Consider incorporating mindfulness practices such as meditation, deep breathing, or mindful eating into your routine to enhance your focus and clarity.

Reflecting on your routine is important for continuous improvement. Regularly assess how your routine aligns with your goals and values. Are there areas that could be optimized or adjusted? Are there activities that no longer serve your well-being? Use this reflection as an opportunity to make positive changes and refine your routine. By regularly evaluating your practices, you can ensure that your routine continues to support your overall wellness and personal growth.

Avoiding Harmful Behaviors

Navigating the complexities of life often involves making choices that can either enhance or detract from our well-being. Avoiding harmful behaviors is a crucial aspect of maintaining a healthy and balanced life. These behaviors, whether physical, emotional, or social, can have far-reaching consequences that impact not only the individual but also those around them. By recognizing and addressing these behaviors, individuals can foster a more positive and fulfilling existence.

Understanding the root causes of harmful behaviors is the first step in addressing them. Often, these behaviors are coping mechanisms for underlying issues such as stress, anxiety, or unresolved trauma. They may provide temporary relief or distraction but ultimately lead to negative outcomes. By identifying the triggers and emotions that drive these behaviors, individuals can begin to address the underlying issues and seek healthier alternatives.

Self-awareness plays a pivotal role in avoiding harmful behaviors. It involves being attuned to your thoughts, emotions, and actions, allowing you to recognize patterns and make conscious choices. Practicing self-reflection through journaling, meditation, or therapy can enhance self-awareness and provide insights into your behavior. By understanding your motivations and triggers, you can develop strategies to avoid harmful behaviors and make more intentional choices.

Setting clear boundaries is essential for protecting yourself from harmful influences. Boundaries define what is acceptable and unacceptable behavior, both for yourself and others. Communicating your boundaries assertively can prevent situations that may lead to harmful behaviors. Whether it's declining invitations to environments that encourage negative habits or limiting interactions with individuals who do not respect your boundaries, setting limits is a powerful tool for maintaining your well-being.

Building a support network is invaluable in avoiding harmful behaviors. Surrounding yourself with positive influences and individuals who support your goals can provide encouragement and accountability. Whether it's friends, family, or support groups, having a network of people who understand your journey can make a significant difference. They can offer guidance, share experiences, and provide a sense of community that reinforces your commitment to positive change.

Developing healthy coping mechanisms is crucial for managing stress and emotions without resorting to harmful behaviors. Engaging in activities that promote relaxation and well-being, such as exercise, creative pursuits, or mindfulness practices, can provide a constructive outlet for emotions. These activities not only reduce stress but also enhance your overall quality of life, making it easier to resist the temptation of harmful behaviors.

Education and awareness are powerful tools in avoiding harmful behaviors. Understanding the potential consequences of these behaviors can serve as a deterrent and motivate individuals to seek healthier alternatives. Whether it's learning about the health risks associated with substance abuse or the impact of negative self-talk on mental health, knowledge empowers individuals to make informed choices. Staying informed about the latest research and resources can also provide valuable insights and support.

Mindfulness can be a transformative practice in avoiding harmful behaviors. By cultivating awareness of the present moment, individuals can interrupt automatic responses and make conscious choices.

Mindfulness allows you to observe your thoughts and emotions without judgment, creating space for reflection and intentional action. Incorporating mindfulness practices into your daily routine can enhance your ability to manage stress and make healthier choices.

Seeking professional help is an important step for individuals struggling with harmful behaviors. Therapists, counselors, and support groups can provide guidance, support, and strategies for change. Professional help offers a safe space to explore underlying issues, develop coping mechanisms, and create a personalized plan for positive change. It's important to remember that seeking help is a sign of strength and a proactive step toward a healthier life.

Celebrating progress and milestones is essential for maintaining motivation and commitment to change. Acknowledging your achievements, no matter how small, reinforces positive behavior and boosts self-esteem. Consider rewarding yourself for reaching goals or overcoming challenges, whether it's treating yourself to a favorite activity or sharing your success with loved ones. Celebrating progress creates a positive feedback loop that encourages continued growth and resilience.

Flexibility and adaptability are important qualities in avoiding harmful behaviors. Life is unpredictable, and setbacks are a natural part of the journey. It's important to approach challenges with resilience and a willingness to learn. Instead of viewing setbacks as failures, see them as opportunities for growth and reflection. By maintaining a flexible mindset, you can navigate obstacles with grace and continue to make progress toward a healthier life.

In the pursuit of avoiding harmful behaviors, it's important to remember that change is a gradual and ongoing process. It's about making intentional choices that align with your values and aspirations. By focusing on progress rather than perfection, you can cultivate a sense of fulfillment and well-being. Embrace the journey of positive change, and discover the profound impact it can have on your life and the lives of those around you.

Embracing Change and Adaptability

Change is an inevitable part of life, a constant that shapes our experiences and challenges our perceptions. Embracing change and cultivating adaptability are essential skills for navigating the complexities of the modern world. These skills empower individuals to respond to new circumstances with resilience and creativity, transforming potential obstacles into opportunities for growth and development.

The journey of embracing change begins with a shift in mindset. Often, change is met with resistance due to fear of the unknown or discomfort with uncertainty. However, by viewing change as an opportunity rather than a threat, individuals can open themselves to new possibilities and experiences. This mindset shift involves cultivating curiosity and a willingness to explore the unfamiliar. By approaching change with an open mind, you can discover new perspectives and insights that enrich your life.

Adaptability is the ability to adjust to new conditions and environments with ease. It involves being flexible in your thinking and actions, allowing you to navigate change with confidence. Developing adaptability requires a willingness to let go of rigid expectations and embrace a more fluid approach to life. This flexibility enables you to respond to challenges with creativity and resourcefulness, finding innovative solutions to problems and seizing opportunities as they arise.

One of the key components of adaptability is resilience, the capacity to recover from setbacks and adversity. Resilience is built through experience and reflection, allowing individuals to learn from challenges and emerge stronger. By cultivating resilience, you can maintain a positive outlook and persevere in the face of difficulties. This resilience is bolstered by a strong support network, including friends, family, and mentors who provide encouragement and guidance during times of change.

Embracing change also involves setting realistic expectations and goals. Change can be overwhelming, especially when it involves significant life transitions or challenges. By breaking down larger changes into smaller, manageable steps, you can create a clear path forward and reduce feelings of overwhelm. Setting achievable goals provides a sense of direction and purpose, allowing you to focus on progress rather than perfection.

Mindfulness is a valuable practice for navigating change with grace and presence. By cultivating awareness of the present moment, you can reduce anxiety about the future and remain grounded in the here and now. Mindfulness allows you to observe your thoughts and emotions without judgment, creating space for reflection and intentional action. Incorporating mindfulness practices such as meditation, deep breathing, or mindful walking into your routine can enhance your ability to adapt to change and maintain a sense of calm amidst uncertainty.

Learning from past experiences is an important aspect of embracing change. Reflecting on previous transitions and challenges can provide valuable insights and lessons that inform your approach to future changes. Consider what strategies were effective, what obstacles you encountered, and how you overcame them. By learning from the past, you can develop a toolkit of skills and strategies that support your adaptability and resilience.

Embracing change also involves being open to new opportunities and experiences. Often, change brings with it the potential for growth and discovery. By remaining open to new possibilities, you can expand your horizons and enrich your life. This openness requires a willingness to step outside your comfort zone and take risks, trusting in your ability to navigate the unknown. Whether it's pursuing a new career, exploring a new hobby, or traveling to a new destination, embracing new experiences can lead to personal and professional growth.

Communication is a crucial skill for navigating change, particularly in collaborative or team environments. Effective communication involves expressing your thoughts and feelings clearly and listening actively to others. By fostering open and honest communication, you can build trust and understanding, facilitating smoother transitions and collaboration. This communication also involves being receptive to feedback and willing to adjust your approach based on input from others.

Self-care is an essential component of embracing change and maintaining adaptability. Change can be physically and emotionally demanding, making it important to prioritize activities that nurture your well-being. Regular exercise, healthy eating, and adequate rest are foundational elements of self-care that support your physical health. Additionally, engaging in activities that promote relaxation and joy, such as hobbies or spending time with loved ones, can enhance your emotional well-being and resilience.

In the journey of embracing change, it's important to celebrate progress and milestones. Acknowledging your achievements, no matter how small, reinforces positive behavior and boosts self-esteem. Consider rewarding yourself for reaching goals or overcoming challenges, whether it's treating yourself to a favorite activity or sharing your success with loved ones. Celebrating progress creates a positive feedback loop that encourages continued growth and adaptability.

Chapter 6
Overcoming Challenges

Dealing with Setbacks and Plateaus

Setbacks and plateaus are inevitable parts of any journey toward personal growth and achievement. Whether you're striving for professional success, personal development, or physical fitness, encountering obstacles and periods of stagnation is a natural part of the process. Understanding how to effectively deal with these challenges can make the difference between giving up and pushing forward with renewed determination.

The first step in dealing with setbacks is to acknowledge and accept them as a normal part of life. Everyone experiences setbacks at some point, and they do not define your worth or potential. By accepting setbacks as opportunities for learning and growth, you can shift your perspective and approach them with a more positive mindset. This acceptance allows you to move forward without being weighed down by self-doubt or frustration.

Reflecting on the causes of a setback is crucial for gaining insights and making informed decisions about your next steps. Take the time to analyze what went wrong and identify any contributing factors. Was it a lack of preparation, unforeseen circumstances, or perhaps an unrealistic goal? By understanding the root causes, you can develop strategies to address them and prevent similar setbacks in the future. This reflection process is not about assigning blame but about gaining clarity and learning from the experience.

Once you've identified the causes of a setback, it's important to adjust your goals and expectations accordingly. Setbacks often require a reassessment of your objectives and the strategies you're using to achieve them. This may involve setting more realistic goals, breaking down larger tasks into smaller, manageable steps, or exploring alternative approaches. By being flexible and open to change, you can adapt to new circumstances and continue making progress toward your goals.

Building resilience is a key component of overcoming setbacks. Resilience is the ability to bounce back from adversity and maintain a positive outlook despite challenges. Developing resilience involves cultivating a growth mindset, which is the belief that abilities and intelligence can be developed through effort and learning. By embracing a growth mindset, you can view setbacks as opportunities for growth and improvement rather than as insurmountable obstacles.

Seeking support from others can provide valuable encouragement and perspective during times of setback. Whether it's friends, family, mentors, or support groups, having a network of people who understand your journey can make a significant difference. They can offer guidance, share experiences, and provide a sense of community that reinforces your commitment to overcoming challenges. Don't hesitate to reach out for support when you need it, as it can be a powerful source of motivation and strength.

Plateaus, on the other hand, are periods where progress seems to stall despite continued effort. They can be particularly frustrating because it feels as though you're putting in the work without seeing results. However, plateaus are a natural part of any growth process and can be an opportunity to reassess and refine your approach.

One effective strategy for overcoming plateaus is to introduce variety and change into your routine. This could involve trying new techniques, setting different goals, or exploring new areas of interest. For example, if you've hit a plateau in your fitness routine, consider incorporating new exercises or changing your workout schedule. By introducing variety, you can challenge your body and mind in new ways, reigniting your motivation and breaking through the plateau.

Another approach to dealing with plateaus is to focus on the process rather than the outcome. Instead of fixating on the end goal, shift your attention to the daily actions and habits that contribute to your progress. Celebrate small victories and acknowledge the effort you're putting in, even if the results aren't immediately visible. This focus on the process can help maintain motivation and prevent feelings of discouragement.

Mindfulness can also be a valuable tool for navigating setbacks and plateaus. By cultivating awareness of the present moment, you can reduce anxiety about the future and remain grounded in the here and now. Mindfulness allows you to observe your thoughts and emotions without judgment, creating space for reflection and intentional action. Incorporating mindfulness practices such as meditation, deep breathing, or mindful journaling into your routine can enhance your ability to manage setbacks and plateaus with grace and resilience.

It's important to remember that setbacks and plateaus are temporary and do not define your overall journey. They are simply moments in time that provide opportunities for growth, learning, and self-discovery. By approaching these challenges with a positive mindset and a willingness to adapt, you can continue moving forward and ultimately achieve your goals.

Managing Chronic Conditions

Living with a chronic condition presents unique challenges that require ongoing management and adaptation. These conditions, which can include diabetes, arthritis, asthma, and heart disease, often demand a comprehensive approach to maintain quality of life and prevent complications. Successfully managing a chronic condition involves understanding the condition itself, developing a personalized care plan, and fostering a supportive environment.

Understanding your chronic condition is the foundation of effective management. This involves educating yourself about the condition's causes, symptoms, and potential complications. Knowledge empowers you to make informed decisions about your health and treatment options. Consult with healthcare professionals, read reputable sources, and consider joining support groups to gain insights and share experiences with others facing similar challenges. By becoming well-informed, you can actively participate in your care and advocate for your needs.

Developing a personalized care plan is essential for managing a chronic condition. This plan should be tailored to your specific needs and goals, taking into account your lifestyle, preferences, and any other health considerations. Work closely with your healthcare team to create a plan that includes medication management, lifestyle modifications, and regular monitoring. This collaborative approach ensures that your care plan is comprehensive and adaptable to changes in your condition or circumstances.

Medication management is often a critical component of managing chronic conditions. It's important to understand your medications, including their purpose, dosage, and potential side effects. Adhering to your prescribed medication regimen is crucial for controlling symptoms and preventing complications. Use tools such as pill organizers, alarms, or mobile apps to help you remember to take your medications as directed. If you experience any side effects or have concerns about your medications, communicate with your healthcare provider to explore alternatives or adjustments.

Lifestyle modifications play a significant role in managing chronic conditions. These changes can include adopting a balanced diet, engaging in regular physical activity, and managing stress. A nutritious diet can help control symptoms and improve overall health. Work with a registered dietitian to develop a meal plan that meets your nutritional needs and supports your condition. Regular exercise can enhance physical function, boost mood, and reduce the risk of complications. Choose activities that you enjoy and that are appropriate for your condition, and aim for consistency rather than intensity.

Stress management is another important aspect of managing chronic conditions. Chronic stress can exacerbate symptoms and negatively impact your health. Incorporate stress-reducing practices into your daily routine, such as mindfulness meditation, deep breathing exercises, or yoga. These practices can help you maintain a sense of calm and resilience, even in the face of challenges. Additionally, consider seeking support from a mental health professional if you experience anxiety or depression related to your condition.

Regular monitoring and follow-up care are essential for managing chronic conditions. Keep track of your symptoms, medication adherence, and any changes in your condition. Use a journal or digital app to record this information, and share it with your healthcare team during appointments. Regular check-ups and screenings can help detect any changes or complications early, allowing for timely intervention. Stay proactive in scheduling and attending these appointments, and communicate openly with your healthcare providers about any concerns or questions.

Building a supportive environment is crucial for managing a chronic condition. Surround yourself with friends, family, and healthcare professionals who understand your journey and can provide encouragement and assistance. Share your experiences and needs with your support network, and don't hesitate to ask for help when needed. Whether it's assistance with daily tasks, emotional support, or attending medical appointments, having a strong support system can make a significant difference in your ability to manage your condition.

Advocating for yourself is an important skill when managing a chronic condition. This involves communicating your needs and preferences to your healthcare team and ensuring that your voice is heard in decision-making processes. Be proactive in seeking information, asking questions, and expressing any concerns you may have. Remember that you are an active participant in your care, and your input is valuable in creating a treatment plan that aligns with your goals and values.

Technology can be a valuable tool in managing chronic conditions. From mobile apps that track symptoms and medications to wearable devices that monitor vital signs, technology can provide real-time data and insights into your health. Explore the available options and choose tools that complement your care plan and lifestyle. These technologies can enhance your ability to manage your condition and provide valuable information to your healthcare team.

Embracing a positive mindset is essential for living well with a chronic condition. While managing a chronic condition can be challenging, focusing on what you can control and celebrating small victories can foster a sense of empowerment and resilience. Set realistic goals and acknowledge your progress, no matter how small. Cultivate gratitude and mindfulness to enhance your overall well-being and maintain a positive outlook.

Injury Prevention and Recovery

Injury prevention and recovery are integral components of maintaining a healthy and active lifestyle. Whether you're an athlete, a weekend warrior, or someone who enjoys regular physical activity, understanding how to prevent injuries and recover effectively is crucial for long-term well-being. By adopting proactive strategies and embracing a holistic approach to recovery, you can minimize the risk of injury and ensure a swift return to your favorite activities.

Preventing injuries begins with proper preparation and awareness. One of the most effective ways to reduce the risk of injury is through a comprehensive warm-up routine. Warming up increases blood flow to the muscles, enhances flexibility, and prepares the body for physical exertion. A well-rounded warm-up should include dynamic stretches and movements that mimic the activity you're about to engage in. For example, if you're preparing for a run, incorporate leg swings, high knees, and gentle jogging to activate the muscles and joints involved in running.

In addition to warming up, maintaining proper form and technique is essential for injury prevention. Whether you're lifting weights, practicing yoga, or playing a sport, using the correct form reduces the strain on your muscles and joints and minimizes the risk of overuse injuries. Consider working with a coach or trainer to learn the proper techniques for your chosen activities. Regularly reviewing and refining your form can help prevent injuries and improve your overall performance.

Listening to your body is a key aspect of injury prevention. Pay attention to any signs of discomfort or fatigue, and don't ignore persistent pain. Pushing through pain can lead to more serious injuries and prolonged recovery times. Instead, take a break, modify your activity, or seek professional advice if you experience pain that doesn't subside with rest. By respecting your body's signals, you can prevent minor issues from escalating into major injuries.

Cross-training is another effective strategy for injury prevention. Engaging in a variety of activities helps balance muscle development and reduces the risk of overuse injuries. For instance, if you're a runner, incorporating swimming or cycling into your routine can provide cardiovascular benefits while giving your joints a break from the repetitive impact of running. Cross-training also keeps your workouts interesting and challenging, which can enhance motivation and adherence to your fitness routine.

Proper nutrition and hydration play a vital role in injury prevention and recovery. A balanced diet rich in essential nutrients supports muscle repair and overall health. Ensure you're consuming adequate protein, healthy fats, and carbohydrates to fuel your body and aid in recovery. Hydration is equally important, as it helps maintain joint lubrication and supports cellular function. Drink water regularly throughout the day, and consider electrolyte-rich beverages during intense or prolonged exercise.

When injuries do occur, a thoughtful and comprehensive recovery plan is essential for a successful return to activity. The first step in recovery is to rest and allow the injured area to heal. Rest doesn't necessarily mean complete inactivity; rather, it involves modifying your activities to avoid aggravating the injury. Depending on the severity of the injury, this may involve reducing the intensity or duration of your workouts or focusing on low-impact activities that don't stress the injured area.

Applying the R.I.C.E. method—Rest, Ice, Compression, and Elevation—can be effective in managing acute injuries such as sprains or strains. Ice helps reduce swelling and inflammation, while compression and elevation minimize fluid accumulation and promote healing. Use ice packs for 15-20 minutes at a time, several times a day, and consider using compression bandages or sleeves to support the injured area.

Physical therapy and rehabilitation exercises are often crucial components of the recovery process. A physical therapist can design a personalized rehabilitation program that addresses your specific needs and goals. These exercises focus on restoring strength, flexibility, and range of motion to the injured area, helping you regain function and prevent future injuries. Adhering to your rehabilitation plan and attending regular therapy sessions can significantly enhance your recovery outcomes.

Incorporating mindfulness and relaxation techniques into your recovery routine can also be beneficial. Practices such as meditation, deep breathing, and gentle yoga can reduce stress and promote a sense of calm, which can aid in the healing process. These techniques can also help you maintain a positive mindset and cope with the emotional challenges that may arise during recovery.

As you progress through your recovery, it's important to gradually reintroduce activity and monitor your body's response. Start with low-intensity exercises and gradually increase the intensity and duration as your strength and confidence improve. Pay attention to any signs of discomfort or pain, and adjust your activities accordingly. Patience and consistency are key during this phase, as rushing the process can lead to setbacks or re-injury.

Building a support network can provide valuable encouragement and motivation during your recovery journey. Share your experiences and progress with friends, family, or support groups who understand your challenges and can offer guidance and empathy. Having a strong support system can boost your

morale and help you stay committed to your recovery
goals.

Navigating Social and Cultural Influences

Social and cultural influences shape our perceptions,
behaviors, and interactions in profound ways.
Navigating these influences requires a keen awareness
of the diverse factors that impact our lives, from
societal norms and cultural traditions to media
representations and peer pressures. By understanding
and critically engaging with these influences,
individuals can make informed choices that align with
their values and aspirations.

Cultural influences are deeply embedded in our
identities and often dictate the way we view the world.
These influences can be seen in language, customs,
beliefs, and values that are passed down through
generations. They provide a sense of belonging and
continuity, yet they can also impose limitations on
personal expression and growth. Recognizing the
cultural narratives that shape your identity is the first
step in navigating these influences. Reflect on the
traditions and beliefs that have been instilled in you
and consider how they align with your personal values
and goals.

Social influences, on the other hand, are more fluid and can change rapidly with societal trends and technological advancements. These influences often manifest through interactions with family, friends, colleagues, and the broader community. Social norms dictate acceptable behavior and can exert pressure to conform. While these norms can foster social cohesion, they can also stifle individuality and creativity. To navigate social influences effectively, it's important to cultivate self-awareness and confidence in your own beliefs and choices. This involves questioning societal expectations and considering whether they truly serve your well-being and aspirations.

Media plays a significant role in shaping social and cultural influences. From television and film to social media and advertising, media representations can reinforce stereotypes, shape perceptions, and influence behavior. Being a critical consumer of media involves questioning the messages and values being presented and considering their impact on your beliefs and actions. Seek out diverse perspectives and voices that challenge dominant narratives and broaden your understanding of the world.

Peer pressure is a powerful social influence that can impact decision-making and behavior, particularly among young people. The desire to fit in and be accepted by peers can lead individuals to engage in behaviors that may not align with their values or best interests. Navigating peer pressure requires a strong sense of self and the ability to assert your boundaries. Practice saying no to situations that make you uncomfortable and surround yourself with individuals who respect your choices and support your goals.

Cultural competence is an essential skill for navigating social and cultural influences in an increasingly interconnected world. This involves understanding and appreciating cultural differences and being able to interact effectively with people from diverse backgrounds. Developing cultural competence requires openness, empathy, and a willingness to learn from others. Engage in conversations with individuals from different cultures, seek out cultural experiences, and educate yourself about global issues and perspectives.

Balancing cultural heritage with personal identity is a common challenge for individuals navigating social and cultural influences. While cultural traditions provide a sense of belonging and identity, they may not always align with personal values or aspirations. Finding a balance involves honoring your cultural roots while also embracing your individuality. This may involve redefining traditions in a way that resonates with your personal beliefs or creating new rituals that reflect your unique identity.

Social and cultural influences can also impact mental health and well-being. Societal expectations and cultural norms can create pressure to conform to certain standards of success, beauty, or behavior, leading to stress and anxiety. It's important to recognize the impact of these influences on your mental health and take steps to prioritize your well-being. This may involve setting boundaries, seeking support from mental health professionals, or engaging in practices that promote self-care and resilience.

Education and awareness are powerful tools for navigating social and cultural influences. By staying informed about social issues, cultural dynamics, and global events, you can make informed decisions and engage in meaningful conversations. Consider participating in workshops, seminars, or courses that explore social and cultural topics. These opportunities can enhance your understanding and provide valuable insights into the complexities of navigating diverse influences.

Building a supportive community is crucial for navigating social and cultural influences. Surround yourself with individuals who share your values and support your journey of self-discovery and growth. This community can provide encouragement, guidance, and a sense of belonging as you navigate the challenges and opportunities presented by social and cultural influences. Whether it's through friendships, mentorships, or online communities, having a network of supportive individuals can make a significant difference in your ability to navigate these influences effectively.

Seeking Professional Guidance

Seeking professional guidance is a crucial step in navigating life's complexities, whether you're facing personal challenges, career decisions, or health concerns. Professionals offer expertise, objectivity, and support that can help you make informed decisions and achieve your goals. Understanding when and how to seek professional guidance can empower you to take control of your journey and enhance your overall well-being.

Recognizing the need for professional guidance is the first step in the process. This often involves acknowledging that you may not have all the answers or resources to address a particular issue on your own. Whether you're dealing with mental health concerns, financial planning, or career transitions, professionals can provide valuable insights and strategies that you may not have considered. It's important to approach this realization with an open mind and a willingness to seek help when needed.

Identifying the right type of professional for your needs is essential for effective guidance. Different challenges require different expertise, so it's important to match your needs with the appropriate professional. For example, if you're experiencing mental health issues, a licensed therapist or counselor can provide support and therapeutic interventions. If you're navigating a career change, a career coach or mentor can offer guidance and resources. Research the qualifications and specialties of potential professionals to ensure they align with your specific needs and goals.

Building a trusting relationship with a professional is key to successful guidance. Trust is the foundation of any effective professional relationship, allowing you to communicate openly and honestly about your concerns and aspirations. Take the time to find a professional who makes you feel comfortable and understood. This may involve meeting with several professionals before finding the right fit. Don't hesitate to ask questions about their approach, experience, and how they can support you in achieving your goals.

Setting clear goals and expectations is an important aspect of seeking professional guidance. Before beginning your work with a professional, take the time to reflect on what you hope to achieve and what specific outcomes you're seeking. Communicate these goals clearly to the professional, and work together to develop a plan that outlines the steps and strategies needed to reach them. Having a clear roadmap can help you stay focused and motivated throughout the process.

Active participation is crucial when working with a professional. While professionals provide expertise and guidance, you are an active participant in your journey. This means being engaged, asking questions, and providing feedback throughout the process. Take ownership of your progress and be open to exploring new perspectives and approaches. By actively participating, you can maximize the benefits of professional guidance and make meaningful strides toward your goals.

Confidentiality is a fundamental aspect of professional guidance, particularly in fields such as therapy, counseling, and legal advice. Professionals are bound by ethical guidelines to protect your privacy and maintain confidentiality. This creates a safe space for you to share your thoughts and concerns without fear of judgment or disclosure. Understanding the confidentiality policies of the professional you're working with can help you feel more secure and comfortable in the relationship.

Evaluating progress and adjusting your approach is an ongoing part of seeking professional guidance. Regularly assess your progress toward your goals and consider whether the strategies and interventions are effective. If you're not seeing the desired results, discuss this with the professional and explore alternative approaches or adjustments to your plan. Flexibility and adaptability are important in ensuring that the guidance you receive continues to meet your evolving needs.

Financial considerations are an important factor when seeking professional guidance. The cost of professional services can vary widely, so it's important to understand the financial implications and explore options that fit within your budget. Some professionals offer sliding scale fees, payment plans, or pro bono services for those in need. Additionally, check with your insurance provider to see if any services are covered under your plan. Being transparent about your financial situation with the professional can help you find a solution that works for both parties.

Seeking professional guidance can also involve leveraging technology and online resources. With the rise of telehealth and virtual consultations, accessing professional guidance has become more convenient and accessible. Online platforms offer a range of services, from therapy and coaching to financial planning and legal advice. These virtual options can be particularly beneficial for those with limited access to in-person services or those seeking flexibility in scheduling.